THE 2003 REPORT OF THE NATIONAL CONFIDENTIAL ENQUIRY INTO PERIOPERATIVE DEATHS

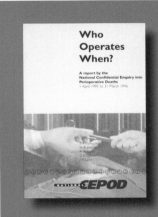

Who Operates When? (WOW I) was published by NCEPOD in 1997. The report defined patterns of surgical activity, placing out of hours activity in perspective.

Compiled by:

M Cullinane PhD (Project Manager)

A J G Gray MB BChir FRCA (Lead Clinical Co-ordinator)

C M K Hargraves BSc RGN DipHSM MBA (Chief Executive)

M Lansdown MCh FRCS (Clinical Co-

I C Martin LLM FRCS FDSRCS (Clinical

M Schubert MSc (Clinical Resea

Published 20 November 2003 by the National Confidential Enquiry into Perioperative Deaths

Epworth House, 25 City Rd, London, EC1Y 1AA

Tel: (020) 7920 0999
Fax: (020) 7920 0997
Email: **info@ncepod.org.uk**
Website: **www.ncepod.org.uk**

Requests for further information should be addressed to the chief executive

ISBN 0-9539240-2-5

A company limited by guarantee - Company number 3019382

Registered charity number 1075588

This report is printed on paper produced from wood pulp originating from managed sustainable plantations and is chlorine-free, 100% recyclable and biodegradable.

Additional information

This report is available for downloading from the NCEPOD website at **www.ncepod.org.uk**

Copies can also be purchased from the NCEPOD office.

The analysis of data from the questionnaires is not included in full in this report. A supplement containing additional data is available free of charge from the NCEPOD office or on the website.

Design and production by Interface, Bristol. Telephone 0117 923 2235

CONTENTS

ACKNOWLEDGEMENTS

This is the fifteenth report published by the National Confidential Enquiry into Perioperative Deaths and, as in previous years, could not have been achieved without the support and co-operation of a wide range of individuals and organisations. Our particular thanks go to the following:

- **The local reporters and contacts for this particular study, whose names are listed in Appendix F.**

- **All those surgeons and anaesthetists who contributed to the Enquiry by completing questionnaires.**

- **The advisors whose names are listed overleaf.**

- **The organisations whose names are listed in Appendix E, who provide the funding to cover the cost of the Enquiry.**

The steering group, clinical co-ordinators and chief executive would like to record their appreciation of the hard work of the NCEPOD staff: Malyun Ali, Philip Brown, Marisa Cullinane, Steven Dowling, Jennifer Drummond, Dolores Jarman and Michelle Schubert.

This work was undertaken by NCEPOD, which received funding from the National Institute for Clinical Excellence. The views expressed in this publication are those of the authors and not necessarily those of the Institute.

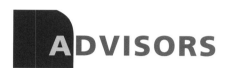

ADVISORS

JS Albert
Consultant Trauma Surgeon
Norfolk & Norwich University Hospital NHS Trust

S Arnold
Site Co-ordinator
Addenbrooke's NHS Trust

R Banim
SpR 3+ Orthopaedic Surgeon
Robert Jones/Agnes Hunt Orthopaedic Hospital NHS Trust

C Barton
Clinical Research Fellow in Orthopaedics
University Hospitals Coventry and Warwickshire NHS Trust

MJ Bell
Consultant Orthopaedic Surgeon
Sheffield Children's Hospital NHS Trust

IP Campbell
Deputy Chief Executive
Bedford Hospital NHS Trust

A Choudhary
Associate Specialist in Orthopaedics
Doncaster and Bassetlaw Hospitals NHS Trust

E Clarke
Group Manager (Surgery)
University Hospital Birmingham NHS Trust

RP Cole
Consultant Plastic Surgeon
Salisbury Health Care NHS Trust

E Cuisick
Consultant Paediatric Surgeon
United Bristol Healthcare NHS Trust

A Curry
SHO Anaesthetist
Norfolk & Norwich University Hospital NHS Trust

PMPD Fernando
NCCG Anaesthetist
King's Lynn & Wisbech Hospitals NHS Trust

AS Garden
Director of Medical Studies
The University of Liverpool

P Gishen
Consultant Radiologist
Hammersmith Hospitals
NHS Trust

J D Green
Consultant Anaesthetist
City Hospitals
Sunderland NHS Trust

D Harrington
SpR 3+ Gynaecologist
Oxford Radcliffe
Hospital NHS Trust

PB Harvey
Consultant Anaesthetist
Plymouth Hospitals
NHS Trust

EF Hoyle
Senior Nurse, Surgery
The Royal Bournemouth
and Christchurch
Hospitals NHS Trust

PAE Hurst
Consultant Surgeon
Brighton and Sussex
University Hospitals
NHS Trust

R Jasinghe
*NCCG General
Surgeon*
University Hospital
Birmingham NHS Trust

S Jones
Quality Manager
HCA International

K Kelly
NCCG Anaesthetist
Altnagelvin Hospitals
Health & Social
Services Trust

J Kendall
SpR 3+ Anaesthetist
Royal Liverpool
Children's NHS Trust

J Lockie
Consultant Anaesthetist
University College
London Hospitals
NHS Trust

S Mackins
SHO Anaesthetist
Swansea NHS Trust

GF Nash
*SpR 3+ General
Surgeon*
North West London
Hospitals NHS Trust

FP Nath
*Consultant
Neurosurgeon*
South Tees Hospitals
NHS Trust

DJ Niblett
Consultant Anaesthetist
Bedford Hospital NHS
Trust

S Nicholson
*Consultant Breast
Surgeon*
York Health Services
NHS Trust

CN Penfold
*Consultant Oral/Facial
Head and Neck Surgeon*
Conwy & Denbighshire
NHS Trust

R Persad
Consultant Urologist
United Bristol
Healthcare NHS Trust

J Radcliffe
Consultant Anaesthetist
University College
London Hospitals
NHS Trust

S Sangera
SpR 3+ Anaesthetist
Sheffield Teaching
Hospitals NHS Trust

A Seymour
Chairman
Patient Liaison Group,
Royal College of
Anaesthetists

M Sinclair
Consultant Anaesthetist
Oxford Radcliffe
Hospitals NHS Trust

G Trotter
*Consultant General
Surgeon*
Maidstone and
Tunbridge Wells
NHS Trust

K Weightman
SHO General Surgeon
The Medway NHS Trust

M Wilson
Theatre Manager
Birmingham Heartlands
& Solihull NHS Trust

FOREWORD

NCEPOD operates under the umbrella of the National Institute of Clinical Excellence (NICE) as an independent confidential enquiry, whose main aim is to improve the quality and safety of patient care. Evidence is drawn from all sections of hospital activity in England and Wales, both NHS and private and we are very grateful to all those who take part, both as assessors, local reporters and as recipients of individual case reporting forms. I would also like to express my sincere thanks to all the permanent staff of NCEPOD for the enormous amount of work and enthusiasm which they put into the production of our reports and without which we could not hope to create such detailed analysis of, and comment upon, clinically related hospital activity.

The first 'Who Operates When?' (WOW I) report was published in 1997 and considerable changes have occurred in the staffing and surgical activity of hospitals since that time. The introduction of the specialist registrar grade under the Calman reforms and the increase in sub-speciality training has meant that many trainees feel less well prepared to take on the general on-call responsibility of a consultant appointment than they did previously. The 'New Deal' on junior doctors hours, which was finally fully implemented in August 2003, has reduced the time available for training still further. In order to achieve 'New Deal' compliance, almost all surgical and anaesthetic trainees are working shifts, either partial or full, which disrupts training and reduces continuity of care for patients.

Consultants are spending more time undertaking emergency and out of hours work for a number of reasons, so that the frequency with which they work in the evenings and at night has doubled since WOW I. An overall increase in consultant and non-consultant career grade (NCCG / SAS) numbers has meant that it is now possible for many hospitals to run a service where the on-call team has no responsibility for elective cases or out-patient clinics. Designated emergency (NCEPOD) theatres are available on a 24 hour, 7 day per week basis in many hospitals, allowing critically ill patients to undergo surgery without undue delay.

Nevertheless, the direct involvement of consultants in out of hours care still seems to be related more to the size of hospital and the number of available trainees, than to a clear strategy to optimise patient care throughout the 24 hour day. While large hospitals utilise trainees to deliver the majority of out of hours work, and medium sized ones employ NCCG staff, in the smaller hospitals, direct patient care is provided by consultants. Perhaps, in the interests of quality of care, the latter model should be used more widely, but if this is the case, then appropriate rest and time off must be provided for consultants in the same way as for trainees. At present, unlike trainees, consultants do not work shifts and, as an ironical result, are often far more fatigued than their junior colleagues whom they are relieving.

This report again reinforces the need for sufficiently robust information and data collection systems in every Trust. Although this is often believed to be primarily necessary for producing accurate activity data, it is becoming increasingly important in clinical governance, risk management and other indices of morbidity and mortality. The frequent criticism from clinicians is that data only flows in one direction and that they can never extract data for critical evaluation of their own practice. Since the key to accurate data entry is to enable the contributors to use it to the benefit of their clinical practice, system design should allow this to be as easy as the production of activity data.

We hope that the advent of Strategic Health Authorities will facilitate a number of the

recommendations in this year's report, particularly those relating to operational issues around theatre usage. The constraints which exist in almost every Trust, around the availability of theatre space and critical care facilities has to be addressed across regional if not national boundaries. This is of particular importance in super-speciality areas such as cardiac, neuro-, vascular and paediatric surgery and, of course involves sufficient numbers of suitably trained medical and nursing staff as much as buildings and equipment. Organisational issues around efficient theatre usage are also highlighted as meriting special consideration.

Many of the issues highlighted in this report produce an interesting dilemma. While direct consultant involvement in patient care has increased to the benefit of patients, trainee involvement has decreased and the cross-cover, which inevitably occurs with shift working, reduces continuity of patient care and opportunities for training. Although this report seeks to examine the standard of surgical and anaesthetic care both inside and outside normal daytime hours, the knock-on effects of this on the training of tomorrow's consultant surgeons and anaesthetists should not be underestimated.

Dr Peter Simpson

Chairman NCEPOD

INTRODUCTION

At the end of the foreword to the 1997 NCEPOD report entitled 'Who Operates When?' Professor Blandy (then Chairman of NCEPOD) and Professor Tindall (then vice-Chairman of NCEPOD) laid down a challenge that the study should be repeated in five years' time. This report details the results of the repeated study. The reasons that were suggested for a possible repeat of the study were to see what changes there might be as a result of the Calman reforms, the introduction of shorter working hours for junior doctors and the promised increase in consultant numbers.

The task of collecting data on all operations performed in a seven day period was daunting for NCEPOD, but it was hoped that the majority of hospitals would be able to provide the information in electronic format to limit the amount of manual processing that would be required. However,

only 34% of hospitals were able to provide the information in a spreadsheet format, which seems symptomatic of a problem that NCEPOD raises year on year – the need for better hospital information systems. Information management in hospitals has a long way to progress and this is highlighted throughout the report by the extent of clearly inaccurate or missing data.

Whilst accepting that surgical practice has changed in the intervening years and therefore definitions of resources and cases have been amended, it was felt important to try and maintain the definitions used in 1997 in order to determine how much the pattern of operating has altered. Early on in this report, a comparison of the key findings is shown. However, throughout the main body of the report, revised definitions have been used to give more detailed information. Detailed explanations of the definitions are provided in the glossary (Appendix B) but the key ones are shown below:

'Out of hours' – 18:00 - 07:59 weekdays and all day at weekends

'Night-time operating' – 00:00 - 07:59 every day.

To help the staff of NCEPOD distil the key findings from the wealth of data collected, advisors were selected from nominations by Royal Medical Colleges, associations and other connected organisations. Two meetings were held which were audio-recorded. The quotations contained within this report are from these meetings unless otherwise stated. The advisors approached the task with energy and enthusiasm considering the amount of data that they needed to digest and they were soon able to distil the definitive points which directed the NCEPOD staff to provide further analysis or to stop pursuing a particular route of enquiry.

It was also useful during the course of this study to forge links with the NHS Modernisation Agency team who were working on improving operating theatre performance [1] and the Audit Commission who were also undertaking a review into the utilisation of operating theatres [2]. Although we are the last of these agencies to report, it is interesting to note that similar issues have arisen in all three reports especially in the area of information systems, data collection and audit; areas vital if hospitals are to understand the pattern of working in their operating theatres.

NCEPOD has been noted for collecting details of deaths within 30 days of a surgical procedure where that procedure has been performed by a surgeon or gynaecologist and this happened again in 2001/02 (Appendix A).

We continue to be concerned about the apparent differences in data, as reported to NCEPOD and to the Department of Health (DoH) in the form of Hospital Episode Statistics (HES), and it is hoped that in the near future a detailed comparative study will be undertaken to review a number of Trusts' returns to both organisations and to attempt to understand why discrepancies occur.

Despite the requirement for hospitals (both NHS and independent) to participate in the work of the confidential enquiries as part of clinical governance, and for clinicians to respond to requests for information as part of the requirements of Good Medical Practice, there remains a number of smaller independent hospitals that have chosen not to participate in our work. Despite the limited number of deaths these hospitals may have, there are still lessons to be learnt and NCEPOD urges them to reconsider their commitment to our work.

This report has been sent to all chief executives and medical directors of NHS Trusts or Independent Hospital Groups with copies for each of their clinical directorates. It has also been sent to local reporters who undertook the major task of co-ordinating all the data collection. Multiple copies of executive summaries have also been sent to all Trusts and Independent Hospitals and the full text of the report can be downloaded from the NCEPOD website **www.ncepod.org.uk** In addition, medical libraries and post-graduate deans are sent copies of the full report.

Christobel Hargraves

Chief Executive NCEPOD

PRINCIPAL RECOMMENDATIONS 2003

- Revise NCEPOD classification to include more specific definitions and guidelines, which are relevant across surgical specialities (NCEPOD responsibility).

- Provide adequate information systems to record and review anaesthetic and surgical activity.

- Ensure that Strategic Health Authorities, together with NHS Trusts, collaborate to guarantee that all emergency patients have prompt access to theatres, critical care facilities and appropriately trained staff, 24 hours per day every day of the year.

- Ensure that all essential services (including emergency operating rooms, recovery rooms, high dependency units and intensive care units) are provided on a single site wherever emergency/acute surgical care is delivered.

- Debate whether, in the light of changes to the pattern of junior doctors' working, non-essential surgery can take place during extended hours.

COMPARISON OF MAIN FINDINGS

* 'trained' was used in WOW I and included staff grades, associate specialists, senior registrars and consultants. Since the era of Calman training we now recognise a surgeon or anaesthetist as being a 'trained specialist' following the acquisition of a certificate of specialist training. It is therefore inappropriate in WOW II to use the term 'trained' for any grade other than consultant.

WOW I	WOW II
54% (24,756/45,806) of all operations during the daytime on a weekday were performed in the presence of a consultant surgeon and 56% (22,286/39,767) in the presence of a consultant anaesthetist.	66% (40,706/61,390) of all operations during the daytime on a weekday were performed in the presence of a consultant surgeon and 62% (35,031/56,831) in the presence of a consultant anaesthetist.
71% (32,489/45,806) of the operations during the daytime on a weekday were performed in the presence of a trained surgeon*, where 'trained surgeon' includes staff grade, associate specialist, senior registrar and consultant. The figure for 'trained anaesthetists', similarly defined, was 72% (28,584/39,767).	79% (48,794/61,390) of the operations during the daytime on a weekday were performed in the presence of a trained surgeon*, where 'trained surgeon' includes staff grade, associate specialist, senior registrar and consultant. The figure for 'trained anaesthetists', similarly defined, was 76% (43,253/56,831).
7% (3,221/45,806) of the operations during the daytime on a weekday and 20% (509/2550) during weekday evenings were performed by apparently unsupervised senior house officers. The related figures for SHO anaesthetists were 9% (3,548/39,767) and 47% (1,150/2,436).	2% (1,133/61,390) of the operations during the daytime on a weekday and 6% (178/3,139) during weekday evenings were performed by apparently unsupervised senior house officers. The related figures for SHO anaesthetists were 4% (2,264/56831) and 25% (735/2,990).
37% (1309/3531) of the emergency procedures during weekday daytimes (08.00 to 18.00 hrs), and 6.3% (148/2346) during weekday evenings (18.01 to 00.00) were performed during sessions scheduled primarily for emergency theatre cases. The overall percentage (08.00 to 00.00) was 25% (1457/5877).	66% (3,273/4,936) of the emergency procedures during weekday daytimes (08.00 to 18.00 hrs), and 82% (1,484/1,812) during weekday evenings (18.01 to 00.00) were performed during sessions scheduled primarily for emergency theatre cases. The overall percentage (08.00 to 00.00) was 70% (4,757/6,748).
51% (182/355) of the participating hospitals had scheduled operating sessions for emergency procedures during the day from Monday to Friday.	63% (184/294) of the hospitals that returned a facility questionnaire had scheduled operating sessions for emergency procedures during the day.
46% (19299/42320) of the routine cases started during the daytime from Monday to Friday were day cases.	46% (28,331/61,390) of the routine cases started during the daytime from Monday to Friday were day cases.

1 STUDY PROTOCOL

Recommendations

Revise NCEPOD classification to include more specific definitions and guidelines, which are relevant across surgical specialities (NCEPOD responsibility).

Provide adequate information systems to record and review anaesthetic and surgical activity.

Ensure the correct ASA status is collected as it is an essential part of the patient assessment and record keeping.

Ensure that the information about hospital facilities is accurate in order to ensure that acute services are efficiently and safely managed.

INTRODUCTION

NCEPOD collected data on 72,343 surgical procedures performed in March and April 2002 and collected from 557 hospitals.

The study protocol was based on the first 'Who Operates When?' (WOW I) study undertaken in 1995/6 [3], which looked at the pattern of surgical activity during a randomised series of 24 hour periods which added up to one week's work for each participating hospital. In this first study, just over 53,000 cases were examined and over 5,000 cases performed out of hours were followed up in more detail.

Slight amendments were made to the method of data collection for this study. In particular, data was collected over a seven day period between 6th March and 16th April 2002. A week was randomly allocated to each participating hospital 3 weeks prior to the start of data collection, when they were sent all the necessary information to complete the exercise. This was to ensure that data not routinely recorded could be collected specifically for the study and also to prevent any changes to the organisation of the theatre rota for that week.

In both studies, data were collected retrospectively via a self-completed questionnaire. For 'Who Operates When? II' (WOW II), the original data collection form was revised and additional fields e.g. 'ASA status' and 'specialty of consultant surgeon' were included (Appendix D).

DATA COLLECTION

In September 2001, chief executives of all relevant hospitals in England, Wales, Northern Ireland, the Isle of Man, Guernsey, Jersey, the Ministry of Defence and the independent sector were asked to identify a person to provide data on surgical procedures to NCEPOD. A letter was sent to Independent Hospitals asking them if they wished to participate.

Chief executives and local reporters of participating hospitals were given the opportunity to provide feedback on the proposed method and the draft questionnaire.

Each participating hospital was randomly assigned a seven day period within March or April 2002 during which to complete questionnaires on all surgical procedures. Data collection was planned to avoid public holidays.

NCEPOD informed the study contact of the relevant week, three weeks in advance of the date. If the contact was unavailable (e.g. on annual leave) they were asked to ensure that there was a replacement contact identified to NCEPOD. The study contact was sent a pack including questionnaires, notes about completion of the questionnaire, and definitions of terms used.

During the designated seven day period, surgeons, gynaecologists and dental surgeons were asked to complete a questionnaire for every theatre case or operative procedure performed within an operating theatre. Specific exclusions included procedures carried out in dental treatment rooms, X–ray rooms, obstetric delivery rooms or theatres, endoscopy rooms and A & E treatment rooms.

Out of hours cases

On receipt of the data, all procedures for which the 'start time of anaesthesia', or the 'start time of surgery', was between 18:00 and 07:59 on weekdays and all day on weekends were designated as 'out of hours' by NCEPOD. These were the time slots that had been designated 'out of hours' in WOW I and therefore for comparative purposes it was important to keep to these time slots. For each of these procedures, an out of hours questionnaire (Appendix D) was sent to the surgeon and anaesthetist involved in the procedure asking them to confirm or amend the starting time, and to state why the procedure was performed at that time.

General data questionnaire

An additional questionnaire requesting information about the facilities and organisational aspects of operating (Appendix D) was sent to the study contact for each participating hospital. They were asked to forward this questionnaire to an appropriate person for completion.

REPORTING

Hospitals were given the choice of returning the data on the questionnaires provided, or electronically using an Excel spreadsheet. Approximately 34% of the cases were submitted electronically.

Letters were sent to medical directors and study contacts two months after data collection reminding them that all outstanding data should be submitted.

All data from the completed questionnaires were input using scanning software. Following data quality checks, the data were imported into an Access database.

Unlike WOW I, OPCS codes were not allocated to each individual procedure as this was felt to be too time consuming and unnecessary for the data analysis. Where individual procedures/diagnoses have been identified for analysis, searching the text fields for relevant keywords has identified these.

DATA QUALITY AND VALIDATION

To ensure the completeness and quality of the data submitted to NCEPOD, a series of data quality and validation exercises were undertaken. NCEPOD staff liaised with the study contacts about omissions or queries in the data. Questionnaires with key fields missing were referred back to the clinician completing the questionnaire with a request that the information be provided. Furthermore, data validation checks were performed once the data had been imported into the database.

Poorly completed fields

> **The ASA status was missing in 33% of cases and the ASA was incorrectly assigned in a number of cases.**

Certain fields on the questionnaires were particularly poorly completed despite detailed definitions being provided (Appendix D). The ASA status of the patient was missing in 33% of all questionnaires returned. Furthermore, we are concerned over the inappropriate assignation of ASA status. 35 cases were reportedly ASA 6 which designates 'a declared brain-dead patient whose organs are being removed for donor purposes', however on detailed investigation only four procedures warranted this status.

Grade of senior anaesthetist and specialty of consultant surgeon in charge were also poorly completed (11% and 13% missing respectively).

NCEPOD classification of operations

> **NCEPOD classifications are not being consistently recorded.**

Inconsistencies were also identified in how hospitals assign NCEPOD classifications (emergency, urgent, scheduled, elective). For example, three apparently similar cases of forearm fractures in eight year-olds were classified as emergency, urgent and scheduled.

NCEPOD therefore undertook a small qualitative investigation via telephone interview of 15 hospitals, in conjunction with the Audit Commission, in order to determine how classifications of urgency of operations were assigned for the WOW II study.

Our findings suggest that discrepancies exist in how NCEPOD classifications are assigned between specialties and hospitals. Many use a different means of classifying urgency e.g. urgent and routine or emergency and elective.

Although most hospitals that were contacted felt that it would be beneficial to use NCEPOD classifications, most had no procedures in place for classifying and recording urgency and timing of operations, and no monitoring systems in place to determine why and when operations were done at inappropriate times. Two hospitals that were contacted did however indicate that the introduction of NCEPOD classifications had reduced the incidence of operations at inappropriate times.

Interviewees expressed a need for definitive guidelines on assigning NCEPOD classification of operations, particularly with regard to appropriate times for operations and clear definitions of emergency and urgent.

Validation of general data questionnaire

In order to attempt to validate the data returned regarding hospital facilities, the NCEPOD clinical co-ordinators visited 27 hospitals, selected at random. We are grateful to all the staff who took time out of their busy programmes to meet the clinical co-ordinators and show them round their hospital facilities.

Twelve data fields were reviewed, to assess the accuracy of data returns.

In most fields, data returns were judged to be accurate. However, in certain fields the data was inaccurate, or had been missing in the original return, but was easily identifiable by the clinical co-ordinators (Table 1.1).

Table 1.1	Results of validation of general data questionnaire		
Question	**Correct**	**Incorrect**	**Not recorded**
Number of surgical theatres (excluding maternity)	13	8	6
Daytime trauma sessions available and staffed	20	1	6
How many trauma session per week?	10	7	7
Daytime emergency sessions available and staffed	21	0	6
How many emergency sessions per week?	6	10	7
Is the recovery area available & staffed 24 hrs/day all week?	16	5	6
If 'no' to above, who would normally recover patients out of hours?	6	0	6
For each recovery bed/trolley space is there a pulse oximeter?	18	2	7
For each recovery bed/trolley space is there an ECG monitor?	17	2	8
Is there a nominated arbitrator to decide clinical priorities?	16	4	7
If 'yes' to above what is the person's professional background?	5	2	8
Does the theatre IT system record grades of anaesthetists and surgeons present?	12	6	9
Total (%) out of 290 possible correct responses	**160 (55)**	**47 (16)**	**83 (29)**

Number of theatres

The greatest discrepancy was from a hospital which actually had 20 theatres but had reported only 13. Many of the inaccuracies related to only one or two theatres, and there was considerable confusion about whether maternity theatres should have been included or not. Discrepancies arising from the inclusion or exclusion of maternity theatres have been treated as correct in the above table.

Daytime trauma sessions staffed

The one incorrect response to this question had indicated that there were no daytime trauma lists, however the clinical co-ordinator established that daytime trauma lists were available.

How many trauma sessions per week?

Three hospitals indicated that they had no trauma lists, and therefore no response was required from them in this field. There should therefore have been 24 correct responses.

Daytime emergency sessions staffed

The clinical co-ordinators commented that in six hospitals, the trauma and emergency lists were timetabled to be staffed by SpR or SHO surgeons and/or anaesthetists. One hospital had introduced five daytime emergency sessions since completing the WOW II return.

How many emergency sessions per week?

Four hospitals indicated that there were no daytime emergency lists, and therefore no response was required from them in this field. There should therefore have been 23 correct responses.

Two hospitals indicated that the number of weekly emergency sessions available had been reduced to accommodate waiting list pressures on elective work.

Is the recovery area available and staffed by dedicated recovery staff, 24 hours a day, 7 days a week?

There were 12 hospitals which either answered 'no' or did not have staffed recovery available 24 hours/day.

For each bed/trolley space is there a pulse oximeter? For each bed/trolley space is there an ECG monitor?

Two hospitals used systems which allowed continuous monitoring including the transfer from theatre to recovery. Three hospitals indicated that there were several different types of equipment in use, which meant that BP cuffs, ECG and pulse oximeter leads were incompatible between monitors in theatre and recovery. It was stated in one hospital that the reason for this was failure by managers to take account of clinical advice about compatibility in favour of cost constraints, during the procurement process. One unit had recently upgraded its recovery monitoring equipment, but the opportunity to incorporate facilities to print off continuous monitoring had been lost, because of a lack of modest funding.

Is there a nominated arbitrator to decide clinical priorities? If 'yes', what is that person's background?

There were only 15 hospitals which indicated that they had an arbitrator. There should therefore be 15 correct responses.

Does the information acquired by the operating theatres about the case also record the grades of all anaesthetists and surgeons present?

Several systems recorded the names of surgeons and anaesthetists, but did not have the facility to record their grades. In some cases, it was possible to link back to a clinician's profile in order to establish the grade of clinician.

Implications for theatre management of incorrect facility information

The data validation exercise for the hospital facility questionnaire demonstrates serious weaknesses in the ability of hospitals to provide fairly simple levels of information about their surgical services.

It is particularly worrying that information, requested from medical directors is inaccurate with regard to basic information such as the number of operating theatres within a hospital.

This begs the question, how can managers plan and deliver an efficient acute surgical service, if they are unaware of the physical resources such as operating theatres, which are available to them?

This exercise also demonstrated a number of other weaknesses, particularly in relation to the incompatibility of monitoring equipment between theatres and recovery. This could significantly degrade the efficiency and safety of patient monitoring between theatres and recovery.

There are inaccuracies in reporting the number of trauma and emergency lists available. Clinical co-ordinators were told that in a number of cases these lists are timetabled to be staffed by unsupervised trainees; this is unacceptable practice.

DATA ANALYSIS

The data were aggregated and anonymised so that individual patients, hospitals and clinicians could not be identified.

Advisory groups

An expert group of advisors was invited to take part in two multidisciplinary advisory groups, where the aggregated data was presented for discussion. The advisors were selected from nominations provided by professional bodies and included surgeons, anaesthetists, nurses, theatre managers and senior hospital management.

The NCEPOD clinical co-ordinators, who directed the discussion around key issues surrounding the data, chaired these meetings. The objective of this expert group was to review the data, identify areas of suboptimal care and provide an overall assessment of the quality of care.

NCEPOD is extremely grateful to the advisors who attended meetings and who provided valuable advice and commentary on the data.

PARTICIPATION

Data were received from 557 hospitals. 205 NHS Trusts, representing 448 NHS hospitals, and 109 independent hospitals submitted data (Table 1.2). Non-participating NHS hospitals are those that are known to have surgical activity and therefore should have responded. The non-participating independent hospitals are those that subscribe to the Enquiry but did not return data.

Table 1.2	Number of NHS and independent hospitals participating in data collection for WOW II		
	Did not participate	Participated (%)	Total
NHS hospitals	33	448 (93)	481
Independent hospitals	51	109 (63)	160
Total	84	557 (87)	641

Participation among NHS hospitals was high with 93% of all appropriate hospitals submitting data. It is not possible to make a direct comparison of the participation rate because the method of determining eligible hospitals was not reported in WOW I.

Reasons for non-participation

NHS hospitals

Of the non-participating NHS hospitals, five were minor surgical units that did not perform any operations during the study week. Other reasons cited for non-participation included administrative difficulties such as "questionnaires lost" and "local reporter unavailable". One Trust, comprising four hospitals, stated that "we started data collection but did not submit the data because the quality of the questionnaires returned was so poor". Despite contacting the medical directors and local reporters with information about the study several times prior to data collection, one hospital reported not knowing about the study. One Trust submitted data after the cut-off date.

Independent hospitals

One large independent group informed NCEPOD before the study started that they were not willing to participate and this accounts for the majority (38)

of non-participating hospitals in the independent sector. Other reasons included "very few procedures, therefore decline to take part", and "no key co-ordinator available".

Out of hours and general data questionnaire response rates

The response rate for the out of hours questionnaire was approximately 65%. This was slightly disappointing as it was felt that these questionnaires provided valuable information for validating and categorising true out of hours procedures.

71% of participating hospitals (395/557) submitted general data questionnaires. The lack of complete facility information for certain hospitals caused some difficulties when comparing surgical activity and resources.

FEEDBACK

Trusts that participated in the study were sent comparative data showing their performance against other Trusts in the same cluster (e.g. Large acute outside London, Acute specialist) [4] *vide infra* Table 2.1 in Chapter 2. Performance was analysed using three of the key performance indicators proposed by the NHS Modernisation Agency in Step Guide to Improving Operating Theatre Performance [1] and one determined by NCEPOD.

The key performance indicators used were:

- Elective theatre performance: Number of day cases as % of all operations performed.

- Emergency theatre performance: Number of emergency theatre sessions each week. (NCEPOD performance indicator).

- Emergency operations out of hours:

  – Number of operations in categories NCEPOD 2,3 & 4 between midnight and 8am.

  – Total anaesthetic plus operating time in categories NCEPOD 2,3 & 4 between midnight and 8am.

(NCEPOD 2 = Urgent, NCEPOD 3 = Scheduled, NCEPOD 4 = Elective).

This was the first time NCEPOD provided feedback to participating Trusts. The response was positive and it is hoped that this feedback process will become part of future studies where appropriate.

Further feedback on the quality of data submitted by each hospital will be sent to medical directors at the time of publication of the report.

OVERVIEW OF DATA

The total number of operations reported to NCEPOD for this study was 72,831 of which 488 were excluded as they did not fall within the sampling frame e.g. obstetric cases. Therefore, the total number of cases on which this study is based is 72,343, with just over 13% being identified as out of hours (9457/72,343). A breakdown of cases is shown in Figures 1.1-1.3.

The additional 18,181 cases reported in this study compared to WOW I are, we believe, a result of NHS participation becoming mandatory (several NHS hospitals declined to participate in WOW I), and more independent hospitals participating in the Enquiry as a whole.

Fig 1.1 Admission type by hospital type

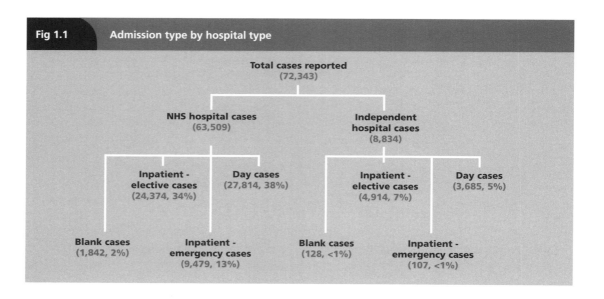

Fig 1.2 Classification of theatre case

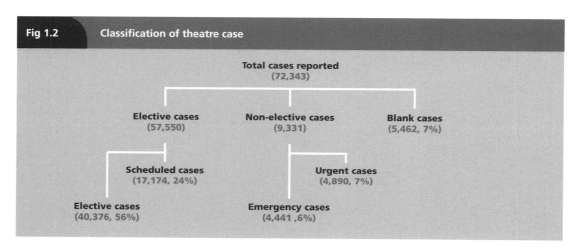

Fig 1.3 Classification of theatre case by hospital type

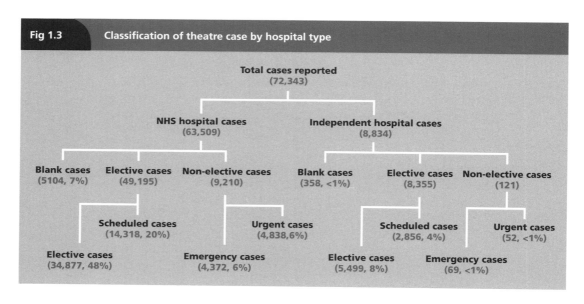

2 FACILITIES

Recommendations

Ensure that Strategic Health Authorities, together with NHS Trusts, collaborate to guarantee that all emergency patients have prompt access to theatres, critical care facilities, and appropriately trained staff, 24 hours per day every day of the year.

Ensure that all operating theatres have sufficient numbers of trained recovery staff available whenever those theatres are in use.

Provide regular resuscitation training for all clinical staff, which is in line with Resuscitation Council guidelines.

Ensure that all recovery bays have both a pulse oximeter and ECG monitor available. This applies whether patients are having local or general anaesthetic or sedation. The equipment used in recovery areas should be universally interchangeable and able to provide a printable record.

Nominate an arbitrator, who would decide the relative priority of theatre cases in order to avoid queuing for theatre spaces.

Ensure that systematic clinical audit includes the pattern of work in operating theatres.

INTRODUCTION

Each participating hospital was sent a general data questionnaire, which asked for details about the size of the hospital and about the facilities available in the theatre and recovery suite. This chapter explores the relationship between the size and surgical capacity of the hospital, and its ability to deliver an appropriate, timely surgical service.

TYPE OF HOSPITAL AND SIZE

The DoH classifies NHS Trusts into 5 main "cluster" groups: acute, multi-service, mental health with community, teaching and specialist. These groups are further sub-divided based upon size and expenditure, with allowance being made for London weighting [4].

Trusts may however be configured in an almost infinite number of ways, and may consist of one large hospital or many small hospitals of different types.

By way of example, Table 2.1 indicates the number of hospitals within the cluster types in this study, and the range of numbers of theatres, as reported to NCEPOD, in the hospitals within the Trust cluster types.

Table 2.1	Number of operating theatres within DoH "cluster" types and range of operating theatres within these hospitals			
Cluster group	**Hospitals**	**Theatres**		
		Min	**Max**	**Average**
Acute specialist	14	1	9	5.0
Acute teaching London	22	1	20	8.5
Acute teaching outside London	52	1	30	8.8
Children's services	4	7	9	8.0
Large acute London	13	1	9	5.2
Large acute outside London	115	1	15	6.7
Large multi-service	18	1	11	5.4
Medium acute London	14	2	16	7.6
Medium acute outside London	78	1	16	8.7
Medium multi-service	28	1	13	6.6
Orthopaedic	4	6	7	6.5
Small acute London	3	7	7	7.0
Small acute outside London	28	1	13	7.8
Small multi-service	14	4	8	6.4

When comparing the ability of hospitals to deliver surgical services, the DoH classification of Trusts has little merit. For example, in a typical city with a population of 300,000, services may be provided by a single site hospital and single Trust, or by several different hospitals at different sites, each providing a different range of specialties, managed by a single or separate Trusts. The DoH classification gives no indication about how acute services are configured.

By contrast, the number of theatres available in a hospital correlates reasonably well with the number of surgical beds (Tables 2.2 and 2.3), and the number of surgical specialties within that hospital (Table 2.4). The number of operating theatres within a hospital is therefore a better surrogate marker of the surgical capacity of the hospital.

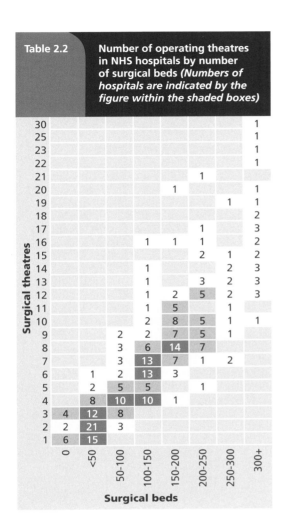

Table 2.2 — Number of operating theatres in NHS hospitals by number of surgical beds (Numbers of hospitals are indicated by the figure within the shaded boxes)

Surgical theatres (rows) by Surgical beds (columns)

Surgical theatres	0	<50	50-100	100-150	150-200	200-250	250-300	300+
30								1
25								1
23								1
22								1
21						1		
20					1			1
19							1	1
18								2
17						1		3
16				1	1	1		2
15						2	1	2
14				1			2	3
13				1		3	2	3
12				1	2	5	2	3
11				1	5		1	
10				2	8	5	1	1
9			2	2	7	5	1	
8			3	6	14	7		
7			3	13	7	1	2	
6		1	2	13	3			
5		2	5	5		1		
4		8	10	10	1			
3	4	12	8					
2	2	21	3					
1	6	15						

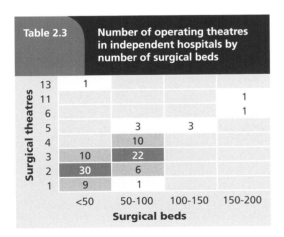

Table 2.3 — Number of operating theatres in independent hospitals by number of surgical beds

Surgical theatres	<50	50-100	100-150	150-200
13	1			
11				1
6				1
5		3	3	
4		10		
3	10	22		
2	30	6		
1	9	1		

Table 2.4 — Number of operating theatres by number of surgical specialties in NHS hospitals

Number of surgical theatres (rows) by Number of surgical specialties (columns)

Number of surgical theatres	1	2	3	4	5	6	7	8	9	10	11	12	13
30										1			
25											1		
23										1			
22										1			
21										1			
20										1	1		
19										1			
18									1	1	1		
17									1	1	1		1
16							1		1	2		1	
15									1	1	2	1	
14								1	2	1	1		1
13						1			1	4	2	1	
12								1	3	4	2	1	2
11								1	2	1	2	1	
10							1	4	4	6	3		
9			1				1	2	4	7	1	2	
8						1	4	8	8	3	6		
7				1	1	3	7	4	6	2	2		
6			3	1	1	1	3	2	3	4	1		
5		1	1	1	1	1	3	1	3				
4	2	2	3	5	6	6	3	3	1				
3	4	4	1	6	3	4	2	1					
2	9	4	7	1	2								
1	5	4	2	5		1							

In the independent sector, the majority of hospitals have less than 100 beds and up to four operating theatres. Unscheduled activity forms a very small percentage (1.4%) of the workload in this sector.

Although a general relationship appears to emerge between the number of theatres and the number of emergency admissions, as reported to NCEPOD, this relationship is much weaker. Whilst in general the more emergency admissions a hospital receives, the more theatres it has, there are some striking variations. One hospital, for example, has 23 theatres, but receives less than 5,000 emergency admissions, whereas hospitals which receive greater than 25,000 emergency admissions, have a range of operating theatres from seven to 30. This may simply reflect the fact that the >25,000 emergency admission grouping is too broad to identify a relationship between much larger numbers of admissions and numbers of theatres. It should also be pointed out that the figure for emergency admissions includes all non-surgical admissions. However, it may be that some hospitals have too few operating theatres to cope efficiently with their emergency workload.

Table 2.5	Number of operating theatres in hospitals by number of emergency admissions					
Surgical theatres	**<5000**	**5000-10000**	**10000-15000**	**15000-20000**	**20000-25000**	**25000+**
30						1
25						1
23	1					
22		1				
21						1
20					1	1
19				1		
18					1	2
17		1			2	1
16				1	2	2
15	1	2			1	1
14		1	1			4
13	1	2		2	1	4
12		2	1		5	4
11	2	3		1		2
10		8	1	5	1	1
9	2	2	2	4	4	2
8	3	6	3	7	6	5
7	12	4	4	2	2	2
6	6	6	2	5		1
5	13	2	2			
4	24	6	2	2		
3	42	4	1			
2	50	1	1	1		
1	27		1			

Emergency admissions

In WOW I it was noted that the proportion of operations which needed to be performed at night in an emergency theatre between Monday to Friday, was 0.5% of the total theatre workload. Taking as an arbitrary starting point the premise that to justify availability of an emergency theatre, one emergency (on average) should be performed each night, this would mean that a minimum of 200 cases should be performed each weekday.

It has already been noted that the optimum catchment population for an acute hospital is believed to be 450,000 to 500,000 [5,6]. The ever-increasing pressure on working hours, so far affecting trainees, will also soon begin to have impact upon consultants.

EFFECT OF HOSPITAL SIZE ON TRAUMA AND EMERGENCY SERVICE

Planned trauma and emergency sessions

NCEPOD has recommended that all acute hospitals should have sufficient staffed emergency and trauma operating sessions, with appropriately trained staff, to permit patients to be operated upon in the timeliest manner [7].

In the 1998 consultation document "Provision of Acute General Hospital Services" issued jointly by the British Medical Association, the Royal College of Surgeons of England, and the Royal College of Physicians of London [5], it was recommended that the ideal hospital should be of sufficient size to provide for a catchment population of 450,000 to 500,000. This consultation document set out several principles, which should govern the configuration of hospital services including the following:

- High quality clinical care, which is timely
- Consistently available sustainable specialist services
- Availability of up-to-date technology equipment and critical care facilities
- 24 hour pathology and diagnostic imaging services
- Optimum training opportunities
- Co-operation between hospitals to give optimum outcomes for specialist or complex conditions.

The ability of a hospital to meet the requirements of a timely emergency service is dependent upon their having sufficient operating theatres. Tables 2.6 and 2.7 compare the number of trauma and emergency lists per week with the number of operating theatres in NHS hospitals.

There is little relationship between the number of dedicated trauma or emergency operating lists, and the number of operating theatres. This is perhaps surprising. It might be expected that those hospitals with a large number of operating theatres would be more likely, by virtue of economies of scale, to provide emergency and trauma sessions every day of the week including weekends. The majority of hospitals have access to trauma lists for five or seven sessions per week with a smaller number having

Table 2.6 — Number of operating theatres by number of trauma sessions per week

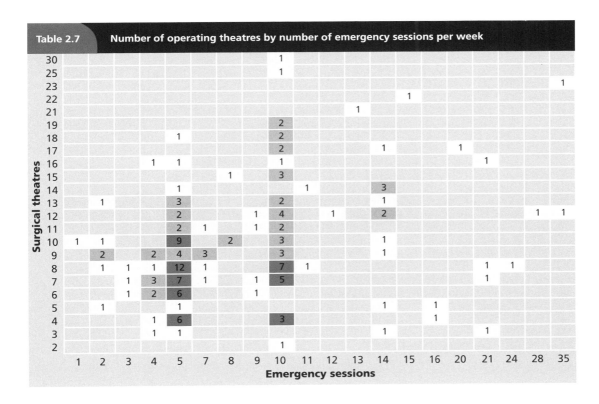

Surgical theatres	0	2	3	4	5	6	7	8	9	10	11	12	14	16	18	19	20	21	27	28
30														1						
25								1												
23							1													
22																	1			
21				1																
20							1	1												
19								1												
18				1				1										1		
17				1				2			1									
16						2		1			1									
15					1		1	1		2										
14					3			1			1									
13				2	2	2	1	1			1									
12			1	3	2	2				3							1			
11					2	2			2											
10				6	3	3			1		1	1								
9			1	7	3	1	1													
8			2	1	12	1	5		2	1	1	3								
7		1	1	2	10	1	3			1					1	1				
6			2		7	1		1												
5		1	1		1	1														1
4		2	1	4	2															
3	1				2															

Trauma sessions

Table 2.7 — Number of operating theatres by number of emergency sessions per week

Surgical theatres	1	2	3	4	5	7	8	9	10	11	12	13	14	15	16	20	21	24	28	35
30									1											
25									1											
23																				1
22												1								
21											1									
19									2											
18				1					2											
17									2		1			1						
16			1	1					1						1					
15							1		3											
14				1									3							
13		1		3					2			1								
12				2				1	4	1		2							1	1
11				2	1			1	2											
10	1	1		9		2			3			1								
9		2	2	4	3				3			1								
8		1	1	1	12	1			7	1						1	1			
7			1	3	7	1		1	5							1				
6			1	2	6		1													
5		1			1							1		1						
4				1	6				3					1						
3				1	1							1					1			
2									1											

Emergency sessions

ten sessions per week. By contrast, emergency sessions are most prevalent for five or ten sessions per week (likely to be weekdays only), with a few hospitals having 14 sessions.

Ideally hospitals that admit emergency trauma should have a dedicated trauma list every day and those that admit surgical emergencies should have an emergency surgery session every day. These sessions should have dedicated, funded sessions for consultant surgeons and anaesthetists, and have the appropriate skill mix of allied health professionals and nursing staff available.

FACILITIES

For smaller specialties and sub-specialties receiving emergency admissions, it may be difficult in small hospitals to achieve the critical mass required to provide dedicated, consultant staffed emergency sessions on a regular basis. Organisation of acute services should plan not only for the larger specialties, but also for the smaller more sub-specialised surgical disciplines.

Whilst the Audit Commission recently identified wide variations in the utilisation of operating theatres between hospitals [2], little mention was made of the need for these theatres to be staffed by appropriately trained surgeons and anaesthetists, together with all the other members of the team, including trained recovery staff. It is likely that despite the modest expansion in consultants, which has occurred in the five years since WOW I, that there will be sufficient trained surgeons to staff emergency and trauma lists in all of the hospitals examined in this study.

The only way to maintain a quality emergency surgical and trauma service is to ensure that there is careful planning and management of resources, so that acute hospitals are of sufficient size to justify the availability of fully staffed "NCEPOD theatres" 24 hours per day seven days per week together with supporting recovery staff. This cannot be achieved in all small hospitals, and is even more difficult to achieve for other surgical specialties where the critical mass must be even larger.

It is too simplistic a solution to state that some hospitals fail to use their theatres efficiently and that the number of sessions left clear to accommodate emergencies should be reduced. True, there may be a case to reapportion theatre time between specialties, and there may be some economies to be gained through this process, but the fundamental problem which needs to be addressed is the organisation of acute services, achieving the balance between scheduled and unscheduled sessions, all of which need to be staffed by appropriately trained medical and allied health professional staff.

This cannot be done by NHS Trusts working in isolation, but needs to be tackled by Strategic Health Authorities.

Recovery staffing

Those NHS hospitals with a larger number of operating theatres are more likely to have dedicated recovery staff available 24 hours per day (Figure 2.1). This is likely to reflect the fact that in a larger hospital, there is a greater number of trained

recovery staff who are available to man theatres on a 24 hour basis. It does not however guarantee that there are sufficient recovery staff available to cover all the operating theatres in use at a particular time.

It is clearly desirable that so far as is possible, patients are recovered by trained recovery staff.

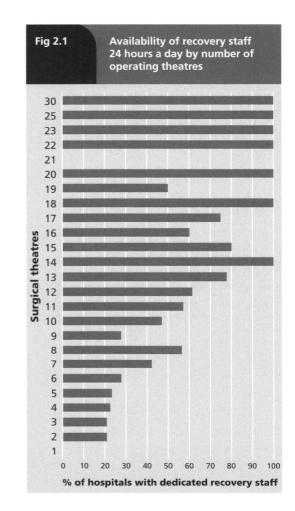

Fig 2.1 Availability of recovery staff 24 hours a day by number of operating theatres

% of hospitals with dedicated recovery staff

Consultant anaesthetist:

"As a consultant anaesthetist of many years' experience…I have never really come across a system which relies upon the scrub staff recovering patients as being as capable and safe as one where you have properly trained recovery nurses. There seems to be a large number of scrub staff who at night recover patients, and I think most people regard that as unacceptable. Recovering patients is a skilled business that should be carried out by staff who not only have proper training but also regularly practice it."

If dedicated recovery staff are not available who is responsible for recovering patients out of hours?

Table 2.8	Staff normally recovering patients out of hours								
	Weekdays			**Saturday**			**Sunday**		
	18:00 - 22:00	22:01 - 23:59	00:00 - 07:59	18:00 - 22:00	22:01 - 23:59	00:00 - 07:59	18:00 - 22:00	22:01 - 23:59	00:00 - 07:59
Dedicated on-call recovery nurse	57	33	26	42	28	25	41	28	25
On-call theatre staff	47	67	74	59	70	76	61	70	75
On-call operating department personnel	2	6	8	5	8	9	5	8	9
Anaesthetist	5	3	4	6	4	4	7	4	4
Other	54	52	52	56	53	51	55	53	51
Blank	140	143	142	140	144	143	140	144	144
Dedicated on-call recovery nurse	19%	11%	8%	14%	9%	8%	13%	9%	8%
On-call theatre staff	15%	22%	24%	19%	23%	25%	20%	23%	24%
On-call operating department personnel	1%	2%	3%	2%	3%	3%	2%	3%	3%
Anaesthetist	2%	1%	1%	2%	1%	1%	2%	1%	1%
Other	18%	17%	17%	18%	17%	17%	18%	17%	17%
Blank	46%	47%	46%	45%	47%	46%	45%	47%	47%

As demonstrated in Table 2.8, out of hours and particularly at weekends, other on-call theatre staff most commonly recover patients. However on a few occasions, anaesthetists were recovering patients.

Consultant surgeon:

" ...it is not appropriate for anaesthetists to be recovering patients."

Consultant surgeon:

" pursuing that point, that also means that the capacity of the theatres is limited because it is always the anaesthetist who is tied up on the next case." sic (should be starting the next case)

Consultant surgeon:

"You cannot run an emergency service out of hours if you tie up your anaesthetists."

In the independent sector, only 19/100 hospitals had dedicated recovery staff available 24 hours per day, and only nine hospitals had more than four operating theatres, so no conclusions could be drawn about the relationship between size and availability of recovery staff in this sector.

Resuscitation training

In NHS hospitals, 93% of responses indicated that recovery staff underwent resuscitation training at least annually. In the independent sector all staff had received resuscitation training within the past 12 months.

However, in the plenary session some advisors expressed reservations about this figure.

Consultant anaesthetist:

"I think there is a protocol in most hospitals that says that they should (have regular resuscitation training) and the managers fondly believe that they do, but we all know that they don't!"

Consultant anaesthetist:

"I am not surprised that the 'yes' response is high. I think that in most hospitals the recovery staff do get resuscitation training but the doctors do not."

Of the 23 consultant surgeons and anaesthetists present at the plenary session, only seven (30%) had undergone resuscitation training within the previous 12 months.

Consultant surgeon:

" I have to admit I have been offered it (resuscitation training), but do we all go?"

Consultant anaesthetist:

" The CNST (Clinical Negligence Scheme for Trusts) requirements are a bit more open minded. They say that the Trust must have a policy about who should receive resuscitation training…. I think Trusts and the general public would expect that all doctors would be competent to at least perform CPR (Cardio-pulmonary Resuscitation) to the level of a 16 year-old St John cadet."

The Resuscitation Council (UK) recommends:

"All doctors should have advanced resuscitation training. Nursing staff should have training to a standard compatible with their level of experience and expected duties within hospital. Ideally, doctors in acute specialties and appropriate nursing staff should hold a valid Resuscitation Council (UK) Advanced Life Support Certificate.

All hospital based resuscitation training should be repeated and reassessed at regular intervals. Training should be valid for a fixed period of time only, with updates recommended yearly as a minimum"[8].

NCEPOD would endorse these recommendations.

Monitoring equipment

In NHS hospitals, 90% had a pulse oximeter and 80% an ECG monitor available for each recovery bay. For independent hospitals, 89% had a pulse oximeter and 85% an ECG monitor for each recovery bay.

The Association of Anaesthetists of Great Britain and Ireland recommends the following [9]:

"Monitoring devices must be attached before induction of anaesthesia and their use continued until the patient has recovered from the effects of anaesthesia.

All information provided by monitoring devices should be recorded in the patient's notes. Trend display and printing devices are recommended as they allow the anaesthetist to concentrate on managing the patient in emergency situations.

Only a brief interruption of monitoring is acceptable if the recovery area is immediately adjacent to the operating theatre. Otherwise monitoring should be continued during transfer to the same degree as any other intra or inter hospital transfer.

A high standard of monitoring should be maintained until the patient is fully recovered from anaesthesia. Clinical observations must be supplemented by the following monitoring devices.

- Pulse oximeter
- Non-invasive blood pressure monitor

The following must also be immediately available

- Electrocardiograph
- Nerve stimulator
- Means of measuring temperature
- Capnograph"

Consultant anaesthetist:

"It is unsafe practice to recover patients without a pulse oximeter or ECG."

Consultant surgeon:

"There might be a situation where there are theatres that are only undertaking local anaesthetic procedures and I would ask my anaesthetic colleagues whether it is necessary to have a pulse oximeter and ECG?"

Consultant anaesthetist:

" I can answer that because the recommendations are that anybody having a procedure under local anaesthetic should have exactly the same monitoring as somebody who is having general anaesthetic."

The Association of Anaesthetists recommends [9]:

"Regional Techniques & Sedation for Operative Procedures

Patients must have appropriate monitoring, including the following devices.

- Pulse oximeter
- Non-invasive blood pressure monitor
- Electrocardiograph"

Theatre arbitrator

In the WOW II study, only 55% of NHS hospitals indicated that there was a designated theatre arbitrator. In the majority of cases this individual was from a medical background (Fig. 2.2).

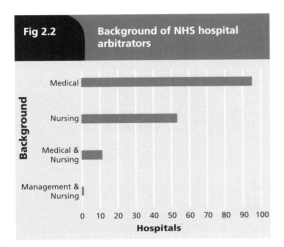

By way of contrast, 81% of independent hospitals indicated that there was a designated arbitrator. In the majority of cases, this individual was from a nursing background (Fig. 2.3).

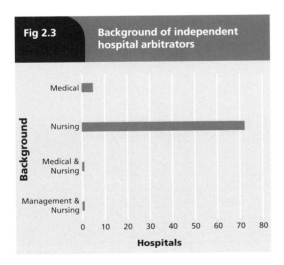

Audit

In response to the question: "Do the operating theatres have clinical audit meetings?" 67% of NHS hospitals indicated that they did, but only 51% of independent hospitals answered in the affirmative.

Of those hospitals undertaking theatre audit, 86% in the NHS and 96% of independents examined the pattern of work in the operating theatres.

Consultant surgeon:

"In many hospitals such as my own, the anaesthetic directorate decides to have audit meetings at which time it withdraws its services. Therefore all elective surgery stops during those times and therefore there is a scheduled audit meeting for everybody. Whether the staff actually attend those meetings is another matter, and I don't think that has been asked."

Manager:

"Unfortunately we all have our own separate audits…the theatre staff audits are the theatre sisters just discussing incidents. We need multi-disciplinary audits, but I am not sure what is the best way to go about them."

Consultant surgeon:

"In the children's hospital we have an audit session at which the whole hospital is supposed to stop working, apart from emergencies. We have consequently managed to have multi-disciplinary audits."

Consultant surgeon:

"In our Trust, clinicians have been trying to push for an all day audit, but the Trust is quite resistant to that because the impact that that would have on its waiting lists and throughput is quite considerable. I would welcome having the opportunity to audit with my anaesthetic colleagues, but it is very difficult unless pressure is put on Trusts to actually insist that they would have time to do it."

Manager:

"I don't think there is such a clear tension between elective activity and audit. First, believe it or not, I think managers do care about the quality of care that patients receive. Secondly, I think even if one was being a bit cynical, if you are going to look at what determines star status, the CHI report is a powerful influence and the CHI inspection will look for good quality audit taking place."

In 34 % of NHS hospitals and 31% of independent hospitals, the grades of the surgeons and/or anaesthetists present during an operation was still not being recorded because hospitals do not have adequate information systems in theatres. This is a lamentable deficiency.

EFFECT OF HOSPITAL THEATRE CAPACITY UPON NIGHT TIME OPERATING

This study has tried to explore whether there is a relationship between the "surgical capacity" of a hospital and the amount of operating out of hours. For each hospital, the total number of emergency admissions per year, was divided by the number of operating theatres. Hospitals were then placed in six bands ranging from 0 - 800 emergency admissions per year per operating theatre, up to 4,200 - 20,000 admissions per year per operating theatre (Figure 2.4). The number of operations out of hours was then plotted in the five most common categories of reason for operating out of hours. As can be seen from Table 2.9, the majority of reasons given justified night time operating on clinical grounds.

Unfortunately, out of the 775 night time operations, no reason was received in 69% of cases. It is therefore likely that the reasons stated in the 31% of responses received are biased toward clinically justifiable reasons. Is it possible that in the majority of cases surgeons were unable to justify operating at night?

The majority of cases were undertaken in hospitals which had a ratio of emergency admissions to theatres of 0 : 3,200. There was no significant difference in the percentage of total surgical cases performed at night depending upon the type of hospital defined by the ratio of emergency admissions to the number of surgical theatres. There does not appear to be any evidence to show that hospitals with a low ratio of theatres to emergency admissions are likely to operate more frequently at night.

Similarly, there does not appear to be any relationship between the surgical capacity of the hospital and delays occurring between admission and time of surgery. However, data were received from only 49% of hospitals regarding delay, and it is therefore difficult to draw meaningful conclusions given such a poor response rate. From the data that we have received however, it is apparent that hospitals of similar size have widely varying degrees of performance with regard to delay. This could be due to variations in staffing levels, or differences in the efficiency of managing services.

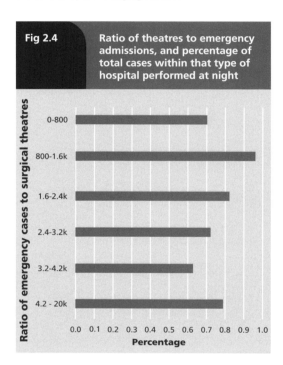

Fig 2.4 Ratio of theatres to emergency admissions, and percentage of total cases within that type of hospital performed at night

As can be seen from Table 2.9, where a response was received, in most cases there was clinical justification for the case being done at night. However, on a small number of occasions, cases were being operated upon at night because there was either no daytime emergency theatre, or the designated emergency theatre slot was over-booked.

Table 2.9	Reasons for night time operating in different types of hospital											
	Ratio of emergency admissions to surgical theatres											
Reason	0-800 (%) n=136		800-1.6k (%) n=92		1.6-2.4k (%) n=100		2.4-3.2k (%) n=59		3.2-4.2k (%) n=7		4.2 - 20k (%) n=3	
Justified on clinical grounds	33	(24)	32	(35)	34	(34)	28	(47)	3	(43)	1	(33)
Daytime theatre already fully utilised	3	(2)	4	(4)	3	(3)	1	(2)	0	(0)	1	(33)
No daytime emergency theatre	3	(2)	0	(0)	1	(1)	2	(3)	0	(0)	0	(0)
Did not need to be done out of hours	0	(0)	0	(0)	1	(1)	0	(0)	0	(0)	1	(33)
Evening/weekend trauma list	0	(0)	0	(0)	0	(0)	1	(2)	0	(0)	0	(0)

GRADE OF SURGEON AND ANAESTHETIST FOR URGENT AND EMERGENCY PROCEDURES

It would appear that the hospitals in the middle of the range of the number of operating theatres are more likely to rely upon Staff and Associate Specialist (SAS) grades both to operate upon and anaesthetise urgent and emergency patients whereas, those hospitals with a larger surgical capacity tend to rely upon either consultants or trainees. Notably, in hospitals with only a few theatres, a high percentage of cases are operated upon and anaesthetised by consultants (Figures 2.5 and 2.6).

Whilst it is perhaps difficult to draw firm conclusions about what these data shows us, what we are able

to say is that there is considerable variation in the patterns of seniority of staff who are available in hospitals with different levels of surgical capacity. In hospitals with large numbers of theatres, most emergency surgery is both operated upon and anaesthetised by either consultants or trainees. This is probably a reflection upon the fact that a hospital must reach a critical mass before there are sufficient numbers of trainees to be available at night. Whilst it is recognised that there is a need for trainees to operate and anaesthetise in the emergency setting, it is also important that "fresh consultants" are available to supervise these trainees, if required to do so.

The hospitals in the middle range seem to rely more upon SAS grade staff. Could this be because they are unable to cover all emergency work whilst also complying with the requirements of junior doctors' hours?

The small hospitals appear to rely much more upon consultants. Do these staff have dedicated sessions for trauma and do they have time off for rest if they have been operating out of hours?

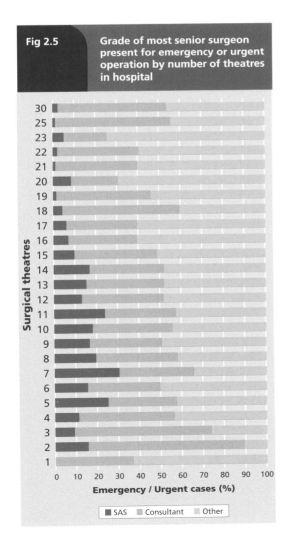

Fig 2.5 Grade of most senior surgeon present for emergency or urgent operation by number of theatres in hospital

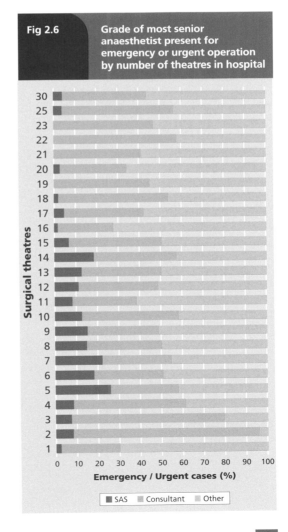

Fig 2.6 Grade of most senior anaesthetist present for emergency or urgent operation by number of theatres in hospital

Recommendation

Assess the competency of staff grade and Trust doctors and take this into account when allocating anaesthetic and surgical sessions.

3 MEDICAL WORKFORCE IN THE NHS

INTRODUCTION

WOW I recommended a repeat of the study in five years' time to see what changes there might be as a result of the Calman reforms, the introduction of shorter working hours for junior doctors and the promised increase in consultant numbers.

Have the numbers of the different grades of staff changed since then and how easy is it to judge the competency of different grades of doctors?

STAFF NUMBERS

> The numbers of staff in post increased between 1996 and 2001 for all grades. The biggest increase, of 124%, was in the number of staff grade doctors.

Data was obtained from the DoH [10] on the number of doctors in post in 2001 and in 1996, by grade and specialty. The data are presented in Table 3.1. Numbers for vascular surgery are included in general surgery because vascular surgery was not considered as a specialty separate from general surgery in 1996.

All specialties saw an increase in consultant numbers. The average expansion was 28% with a range from 3% in oral and maxillofacial surgery to 68% in paediatric surgery. The expansion in training grades has been smaller, with the number of SHOs virtually unchanged and an increase of 16% in

registrar numbers. The number of staff grade doctors has risen from 891 to 1992, an increase of 124%.

NCEPOD decided not to collect data on vacancies because any data obtained would not be meaningful. The DoH does not regard consultant posts as vacant until they have been advertised and unfilled for three months. The advisors had evidence of potential consultant vacancies that were not advertised when there was no prospect of an appointable candidate applying. No information was available for trainee doctor vacancies.

Proportions of SAS doctors and trainees per specialty

Table 3.2 shows the proportions of each staff group as a percentage of the consultant numbers in each specialty in 2001, using the data from the DoH shown in Table 3.1. There was considerable variation between specialties.

Table 3.1	Doctors in post									
							Non consultant career grades			
Specialty	Consultants		Registrars		SHOs		Associate specialists		Staff grades	
	1996	2001	1996	2001	1996	2001	1996	2001	1996	2001
Anaesthetics	2620	3549	1470	1652	1219	1304	206	219	283	592
Cardiothoracic surgery	154	204	165	209	139	152	2	4	10	29
General surgery	1143	1389	677	772	866	938	72	97	94	240
Neurosurgery	124	152	113	134	119	117	1	1	3	16
Obstetrics & Gynaecology	982	1219	863	950	1501	1318	74	87	146	281
Ophthalmology	564	683	309	359	419	398	123	144	90	222
Oral & Maxillofacial surgery	248	256	117	98	339	342	40	49	44	124
Otolaryngology	411	459	197	205	364	355	52	66	54	107
Paediatric surgery	68	114	46	69	98	86	2	1	2	9
Plastic surgery	143	198	117	165	139	157	6	13	11	21
Trauma and Orthopaedic surgery	992	1267	606	823	944	1032	113	131	126	270
Urology	315	427	162	204	152	207	12	25	28	81
Total	**7764**	**9917**	**4842**	**5640**	**6299**	**6406**	**703**	**837**	**891**	**1992**

Table 3.2 Grade of doctor by specialty	Consultants	% SAS	% Registrar	% SHO
Anaesthetics	3549	22.9	46.5	36.7
Cardiothoracic surgery	204	16.2	102.5	74.5
General surgery	1389	24.3	55.6	67.5
Neurosurgery	152	11.2	88.2	77.0
Obstetrics & Gynaecology	1219	30.2	77.9	108.1
Ophthalmology	683	53.6	52.6	58.3
Oral and Maxillofacial surgery	256	67.6	38.3	133.6
Otolaryngology	459	37.7	44.7	77.3
Paediatric surgery	114	8.8	60.5	75.4
Plastic surgery	198	17.2	83.3	79.3
Trauma and Orthopaedic surgery	1267	31.6	65.0	81.5
Urology	427	24.8	47.8	48.5
Total	**9917**	**28.5**	**56.9**	**64.6**

The numbers of staff available in the various grades would have affected the amount and proportion of service work done by each grade in a particular specialty.

Locum doctors

One of the questions asked by NCEPOD for each operation was whether the senior surgeon present was acting as a locum. Table 3.3 shows the percentage of patients operated on when the surgeon was or was not a locum, for each grade of surgeon, for NHS hospitals (no such question was asked about the most senior anaesthetist present). The responses relate to the number of patients, not the number of surgeons.

Table 3.3 Locum surgeons by grade	Was the surgeon a locum?		
Grade of surgeon	% Yes	% No	% Blank
Consultant	6.9	85.5	7.7
SAS	5.6	89.1	5.2
SpR 3 and above	3.7	92.0	4.3
SpR 1/2	6.7	83.5	9.7
SHO	5.2	85.0	9.8
Other	7.2	76.3	16.5
Blank	5.7	46.7	47.6
Total	**6.4**	**83.9**	**9.7**

Factors affecting the availability of trainee doctors for service work

The ability to change the proportion of clinical work done by trainee doctors will be affected by the increase in numbers of trained and trainee doctors detailed in Table 3.1 above. The volume of service work that the trainee workforce can do is also influenced by other factors. NCEPOD has found it difficult to measure the effect of these factors.

A series of initiatives have reduced the hours worked by trainee doctors, but the DoH was unable to supply any figures on the overall reduction in the hours worked by trainees.

Trainee doctors divide their time between educational and service commitments. More of trainees' hours may now be allocated to educational activities than in 1995/96. There are no data to quantify the effect of such a change, and the impact may vary between specialties.

The Calman reforms have led to a reduction in the length of training for doctors. Together with the reduction in hours worked, this can mean that a trainee of a particular grade is less competent to carry out procedures than in the past; for example, it was the opinion of the advisors that the competency of a SpR 1 in 2001 was equivalent to that of an experienced SHO in 1995/96.

COMPETENCY OF GRADES OF STAFF

> **The title of a doctor's post may not be sufficient to judge whether the doctor has the skills to care for a particular patient.**

Several tables in this report compare the grade of doctor caring for a patient with the patient's ASA status. It is assumed as evident that inexperienced trainees should not be caring for the sickest patients, that is, patients assessed as ASA 4 or 5. Conversely it is assumed as evident that the involvement of a consultant guarantees that the care will be satisfactory. The advisors considered that it was not always possible to judge from the title of the post held by a doctor whether that doctor had sufficient training and experience to care for a particular patient.

Trainee grades

As noted above, the competencies of trainee doctors may be less than might have been expected from their grade in the past. However, medical royal colleges are moving towards more structured training. This means that the competencies that a trainee should display at a particular stage of their training are closely defined. There should be no difference in the competency of, for example, a SpR 2 in one hospital compared to another.

Staff grade doctors, associate specialists and trust doctors

There are published criteria of eligibility for appointment to the grades of associate specialist and staff grade. If these are adhered to, then one can be assured that an associate specialist has had a significant level of experience at the registrar level. The criteria for appointment to the post of staff grade are less stringent. Some staff grade doctors may be as experienced as an associate specialist, others may have had relatively little experience and taken up appointment as a staff grade directly from the SHO grade. The post of Trust doctor is unregulated, so that it is impossible to make any judgement on whether it is appropriate or not for a doctor in such a post to be carrying out the work that they are

doing. Whatever their competency when appointed, doctors in these posts will continue to extend their capabilities as time passes, by virtue of continuing professional development and increasing experience.

Given that this group of doctors encompasses such a diverse range of abilities it is not possible to make any overall comment about whether or not a particular pattern of practice for SAS doctors is appropriate. Because of this diversity of abilities, it is essential that Trusts assess the competency of each doctor in these posts on an individual basis. SAS doctors should be allowed to make full use of their talents but should not be expected to provide care that is beyond their capabilities.

Consultants

As one of the advisors observed:

> **Consultant anaesthetist:**
>
> *"I am not sure that the assumption that consultant equals good, both surgically and anaesthetically, is in fact the truth any more."*

Sub-specialisation amongst consultants is common, which improves the care for elective patients, but if the consultant covers a wider range of patients for emergency work, non-elective patients may suffer. On some occasions, this is explicit; a surgeon may specialise on colorectal work by day, with no involvement in the care of vascular patients, but be responsible for ruptured aortic aneurysms out of hours. Sometimes, the deficiency is not so obvious; a consultant anaesthetist may nominally cover general duties, but have little recent experience of upper airway problems. Many consultants, both anaesthetists and surgeons, are gaining little exposure to the care of young children.

It may be difficult to find a solution when a consultant does not feel fully competent to handle a clinical case. In some cases the problem can be solved by the attendance of a consultant who is not on-call. In others, a consultant may decide on the management plan, but an experienced specialist registrar may be the better person to perform a particular procedure than the consultant.

The issue of whether there is a minimum or optimal size of hospital for taking emergency cases is considered elsewhere in the chapter discussing facilities.

THE WORK PATTERNS OF DOCTORS

Most of the tables and figures elsewhere in this report consider staffing issues from the perspective of the patient or the hospital; for example, what are the chances that the surgeon will be a consultant for an elective patient during the daytime on a weekend? It is useful to look also at the data from the viewpoint of the doctor.

Anaesthesia

All cases, elective and non-elective

Figure 3.1 shows the theatre workload of each grade of anaesthetist that was done at each time of the week (workload for each grade defined as the total number of cases where the most senior anaesthetist present was of that grade).

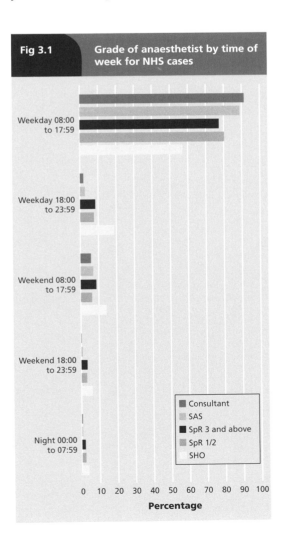

Trainees, and some SAS doctors, will have spent further time in theatre accompanying consultants as part of training or professional development. For all grades of anaesthetist, most of the elective work was carried out during the daytime during the week. This did not apply to non-elective work.

Non-elective work

Figure 3.2 shows the theatre non-elective workload of each grade of anaesthetist that was done at each time of the week (workload for each grade defined as the total number of cases where the most senior anaesthetist present was of that grade).

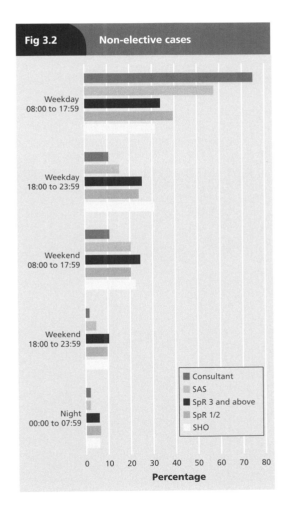

Looking at non-elective work only, consultants did 75% of their non-elective work during office hours, whereas trainees carried out 60% to 70% of the emergency work that they did <u>outside</u> office hours.

It is not possible to tell from the data collected for this report how much teaching on the management of non-elective cases trainees received by accompanying more senior anaesthetists or when this experience was gained. However, it is possible to say that trainees gained most of their experience in anaesthetising non-elective cases on their own when working outside of office hours.

Surgery

All cases, elective and non-elective

Figure 3.3 shows the total theatre workload of each grade of surgeon that was done at each time of the week (workload for each grade defined as the total number of cases where the most senior surgeon present was of that grade).

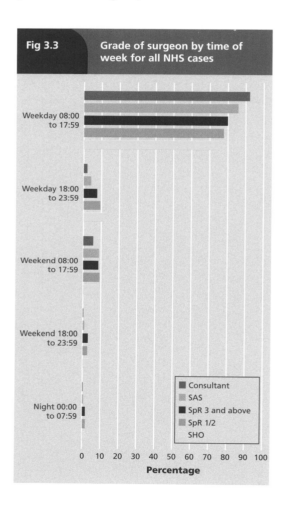

Consultant surgeons did the greatest proportion of their total workload during office hours and SHO surgeons the least, with the position reversed on weekday evenings, but the differences were not large.

Non-elective work

Figure 3.4 shows the non-elective theatre workload of each grade of surgeon that was done at each time of the week (workload for each grade defined as the total number of cases where the most senior surgeon present was of that grade).

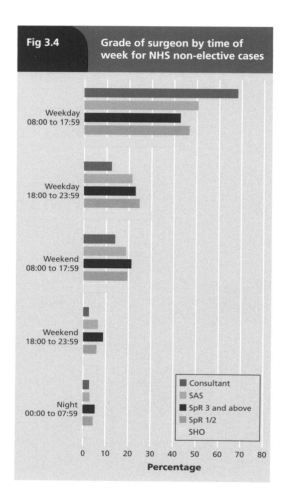

Consultant surgeons did over two-thirds of their non-elective operating during office hours. In contrast, trainees spent only about 40% of their time as the most senior surgeon for non-elective cases operating during office hours.

4 THE PATTERN OF WORK IN INDEPENDENT HOSPITALS AND COMPARISONS WITH THE NHS

INTRODUCTION

This section looks at the general characteristics of all the operations in independent hospitals, with comparisons with NHS hospitals as appropriate. There were 8,834 operations reported from independent hospitals and 63,509 from NHS hospitals.

THE AGE AND PHYSICAL STATUS OF PATIENTS

> Patients in independent hospitals had a different distribution of age and ASA statuses than NHS patients.

Figure 4.1 illustrates the number of operations occurring in different age groups in independent and NHS hospitals.

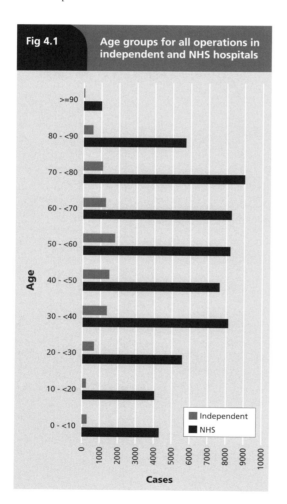

| Fig 4.1 | Age groups for all operations in independent and NHS hospitals |

The age distributions were different. In independent hospitals the largest group of patients was aged between 50 and 59 years, whereas in NHS hospitals, the largest group was aged between 70 and 79. In independent hospitals there were relatively small numbers of patients at the extremes of age, in contrast to the more even spread of the age of patients in the NHS.

Table 4.1 shows the number of patients recorded for each ASA status, for patients in both independent and NHS hospitals.

Table 4.1	ASA status of patients (all operations)			
ASA status	Independent (%) n=8834		NHS (%) n=63509	
1	4946	(56.0)	21747	(34.2)
2	1576	(17.8)	13477	(21.2)
3	313	(3.5)	5516	(8.7)
4	19	(0.2)	881	(1.4)
5	5	(0.1)	146	(0.2)
6	3	(<0.1)	32	(0.1)
Blank	1972	(22.3)	21710	(34.2)

Allowance has to be made for the large number of patients for whom no ASA status was reported, but there was a definite trend for patients in independent hospitals to have a better ASA rating. Independent and NHS hospitals have different proportions of non-elective operations (Table 4.3). If the figures are re-calculated for elective operations only, the pattern is unchanged.

SURGICAL SPECIALTY AND ELECTIVE OPERATIONS

> There were very few non-elective operations in independent hospitals.

The data have been analysed to examine whether the surgical specialties are represented differently in the two sectors.

Table 4.2 shows the number of patients under the care of the different surgical specialties. A greater proportion of the work in independent hospitals came from orthopaedic surgeons than in the NHS. Very few paediatric surgical operations were performed in the independent sector.

Table 4.2	Surgical specialty of operation			
Surgical specialty	Independent (%) n=8834		NHS (%) n=63509	
Accident and Emergency	0	(0.0)	87	(0.1)
Cardiac/Thoracic/Cardiothoracic	165	(1.9)	1020	(1.6)
General	1369	(15.5)	10117	(15.9)
Gynaecology/Obstetrics	954	(10.8)	7639	(12.0)
Neurosurgery	81	(0.9)	608	(1.0)
Ophthalmology	781	(8.8)	6456	(10.2)
Oral & Maxillofacial	303	(3.4)	2206	(3.5)
Orthopaedic & Trauma	2062	(23.3)	10847	(17.1)
Other	274	(3.1)	1367	(2.2)
Otorhinolaryngology	689	(7.8)	4785	(7.5)
Paediatrics	25	(0.3)	771	(1.2)
Plastic	465	(5.3)	2652	(4.2)
Transplantation	0	(0.0)	96	(0.2)
Urology	727	(8.2)	5000	(7.9)
Vascular	181	(2.0)	1322	(2.1)
Blank	758	(8.6)	8536	(13.4)

Table 4.3	Proportion of operations that were non-elective by specialty				
Surgical specialty	Independent			NHS	
	Elective n=8355	Non-elective (%) n=121		Elective n=49195	Non-elective (%) n=9210
Accident and Emergency	0	0 (0)		65	10 (13.3)
Cardiac/Thoracic/Cardiothoracic	160	4 (2.4)		802	165 (17.1)
General	1304	28 (2.1)		7470	2008 (21.2)
Gynaecology	910	23 (2.5)		6172	921 (13.0)
Neurosurgery	79	0 (0.0)		390	165 (29.7)
Ophthalmology	761	3 (0.4)		5984	165 (2.7)
Oral & Maxillofacial	292	4 (1.4)		1899	179 (8.6)
Orthopaedic & Trauma	1977	27 (1.3)		7547	2632 (25.9)
Other	249	2 (0.8)		1054	148 (12.3)
Otorhinolaryngology	669	6 (0.9)		4209	221 (5.0)
Paediatrics	19	0 (0.0)		558	191 (25.5)
Plastic	448	10 (2.2)		1841	627 (25.4)
Transplantation	0	0 (0.0)		66	25 (27.5)
Urology	694	5 (0.7)		4493	188 (4.0)
Vascular	173	4 (2.3)		962	291 (23.2)
Blank	620	5 (0.8)		5683	1274 (18.3)

Table 4.3 shows the orientation of independent hospitals towards elective surgery.

WHEN WERE ELECTIVE OPERATIONS PERFORMED?

Independent hospitals worked a more extended week for elective patients than NHS hospitals.

Figure 4.2 shows the distribution of elective operations across the days of the week (for each sector the percentage bars add up to 100%).

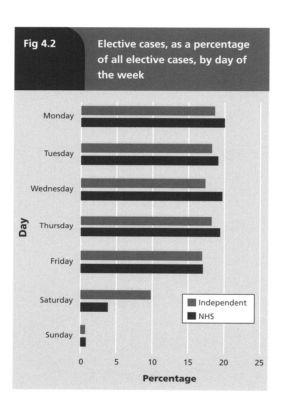

| Fig 4.2 | Elective cases, as a percentage of all elective cases, by day of the week |

The numbers of operations done in independent hospitals were approximately the same for each weekday. In the NHS fewer operations were done on a Friday than on other weekdays. Further analysis showed that the reduction was more marked in the afternoon than the morning. The chart also shows that proportionately more operations were done on a Saturday in independent hospitals than was the case in NHS hospitals.

Table 4.4	Time of day operations were performed			
	Independent (%) n=8355		**NHS (%)** n=49195	
Day	7355	(88.0)	47976	(97.5)
Evening	842	(10.1)	405	(0.8)
Night	116	(1.4)	86	(0.2)
Blank	42	(0.5)	728	(1.5)

10% of elective operations in independent hospitals commenced in the evening compared with 1% in NHS hospitals (Table 4.4).

The working day for elective operations now extends beyond office hours on weekdays for both the private and public sectors. The pattern of a greater extension of the working day in independent hospitals substantiates the common perception that much private operating takes place once consultants have finished their NHS work, in periods when they might otherwise be pursuing recreational activities. There are tight controls on the working hours of trainee doctors in the NHS who are relatively youthful. There are no controls over consultants' hours of work.

FATIGUE

There is a concern that fatigue amongst doctors may lead to medical errors. Attention is usually directed at the impact of lack of sleep, but there may be an effect from working long daytime shifts. Multiple studies [11,12,13,14,15] have documented the impact of fatigue on medical personnel performance. However, these studies have been limited by poor study designs or outcomes that may not correlate well with medical error. Similarly, there are conflicting studies as to whether or not limiting the hours of trainee doctors leads to more errors because of less continuity of patient care. There have also been concerns that doctors may be more likely to be involved in road accidents when driving if deprived of sleep.

Perhaps a more detailed analysis of the risks and benefits associated with limiting working hours should be undertaken, particularly in relation to the deleterious effects on doctors' performance caused by fatigue against the disturbance of continuity of patient care.

DAY CASE SURGERY

Recommendations

Review guidance on which staff should anaesthetise and operate on day case patients.

Review the level of supervision of trainee anaesthetists working on their own in dedicated day case units.

5 DAY CASE SURGERY

INTRODUCTION

Day case surgery is a major part of hospital services. 52% of the elective operations in this report were managed as day cases. It is over ten years since it became accepted that large numbers of surgical patients could be treated without an overnight stay in hospital so it is timely to examine whether care is being delivered to appropriate and acceptable standards.

THE ROLE OF DAY CASE UNITS IN THE PROVISION OF ELECTIVE SURGERY

> **Only 40% of NHS day case patients were treated in a dedicated day case facility.**

Table 5.1 shows, for elective operations, how many patients were admitted as day cases, and how many as inpatients, for both independent and NHS hospitals. The percentage of the total elective workload made up of day cases is also shown.

In 1998, 93% of Trusts carrying out day surgery had at least one dedicated day case unit [16]. NCEPOD asked hospitals to report whether an operation had been performed in a dedicated day case unit or elsewhere. Despite the growth in day surgery, only 40% of NHS day cases were done in a dedicated day case unit and 2% of independent cases were in dedicated units.

Dedicated day case units should have protocols for the preoperative assessment of patients [17,18,19].

These protocols assess whether the patient's social circumstances are suitable for them to be treated as a day patient, and ensure that any extra requirements for nursing and other care, consequent on being treated as a day case, can be put in place. Furthermore, these protocols assess whether the patient is likely to suffer complications postoperatively because of concurrent medical problems. If these assessments result in a judgement that it is inadvisable for the patient to be treated as a day case then the patient can be referred back to the surgical consultant for care to be arranged as an inpatient. Dedicated day units are also likely to have guidelines for the management of anaesthesia and the provision of postoperative analgesia.

Patients booked to be managed as day cases outside dedicated day units may bypass the protection of these assessment protocols unless the Trust has protocols in place for the assessment of day cases managed from inpatient beds and appearing on inpatient operating lists. Moreover they may be cared for by medical and nursing staff who are not used to looking after patients who will be discharged from hospital shortly after surgery. Such patients can be vulnerable to avoidable postoperative problems. Trusts should ensure that all day case patients receive the same standard of preoperative assessment, intraoperative care and postoperative support, whether they are managed in a dedicated day case unit or elsewhere in the hospital.

Table 5.1	Day cases by specialty					
	Independent			**NHS**		
	Day case	Inpatient - elective	Day case %	Day case	Inpatient - elective	Day case %
Accident and Emergency	0	0	0.0	70	9	88.6
Cardiac/Thoracic/ Cardiothoracic	23	137	14.4	52	806	6.1
General	472	853	35.6	3529	4274	45.2
Gynaecology	444	482	47.9	4095	2528	61.8
Neurosurgery	3	78	3.7	22	355	5.8
Ophthalmology	525	239	68.7	5244	996	84.0
Oral & Maxillofacial	199	101	66.3	1456	529	73.4
Orthopaedic & Trauma	753	1261	37.4	3200	4462	41.8
Otorhinolaryngology	195	471	29.3	1462	3019	32.6
Paediatrics	14	11	56.0	253	258	49.5
Plastic	195	249	43.9	1176	731	61.7
Transplantation	0	0	0.0	8	58	12.1
Urology	335	379	46.9	2382	2231	51.6
Vascular	33	143	18.8	386	627	38.1
Other	189	83	69.5	770	358	68.3
Blank	305	427	41.7	3709	3133	54.2
Total	**3685**	**4914**	**42.9**	**27814**	**24374**	**53.3**

WHO IS PROVIDING THE SERVICE FOR DAY SURGERY?

Non-consultant staff cared for more than 40% of day case patients.

The staff performing day surgery in the independent sector will be fully trained independent practitioners.

In the NHS it is recommended that patients undergoing day surgery should be treated by experienced personnel. Guidelines for Day Case Surgery (Royal College of Surgery) [18] states:

"The high standards required demand that both the operator and the anaesthetist must be experienced in the practice of day surgery. Junior trainees should be personally and closely supervised by experienced staff."

Guidelines for the Provision of Anaesthetic Services (Royal College of Anaesthetists) [19]states:

"For this work, anaesthetic involvement must be by experienced personnel working on a regular basis."

"Anaesthesia for day surgery should be a consultant-based service."

"The non-consultant career grades… may provide anaesthesia for day surgery. They require supervision by consultant anaesthetists."

The data returned to NCEPOD have been analysed to explore whether Trusts were implementing these guidelines for day case surgery, and whether patient selection was satisfactory.

Anaesthetics

Table 5.2 shows the number of anaesthetists of each grade caring for day case patients in the NHS, and that number expressed as a percentage of all day cases when an anaesthetist was present. Of the total number of day cases (27,814), 4,853 gave no grade of anaesthetist and in 3,855 no anaesthetist was present.

Table 5.3 shows the number of anaesthetists of each grade caring for day case patients in the NHS divided amongst each location where day patients were treated.

Table 5.2	Grade of anaesthetist caring for NHS day case patients
Grade of anaesthetist	**Number (%)** **n=23959**
Consultant	12092 (50.5)
SAS	3834 (16.0)
SpR 3 and above	779 (3.3)
SpR 1/2	576 (2.4)
SHO	652 (2.7)
Other	1173 (4.9)
Blank	4853 (20.3)

Table 5.3	Location of procedure and grade of anaesthetist for NHS day case patients			
Grade of anaesthetist	**Location of procedure**			
	Theatre suite	**Day case unit**	**Other**	**Blank**
Consultant	6785	4292	338	677
SAS	2067	1527	67	173
SpR 3 and above	455	274	26	24
SpR 1/2	326	205	21	24
SHO	419	181	20	32
Other	535	548	16	74
Blank	1828	2313	250	462
Total	**12415**	**9340**	**738**	**1466**

Surgery

Table 5.4 shows the number of surgeons of each grade caring for day case patients in the NHS, and that number expressed as a percentage of all day cases.

Table 5.4	Grade of surgeon caring for NHS day case patients
Grade of surgeon	**Number (%)** **n=27814**
Consultant	15960 (57.4)
SAS	4958 (17.8)
SpR 3 and above	1881 (6.8)
SpR 1/2	1106 (4.0)
SHO	706 (2.5)
Other	1938 (7.0)
Blank	1265 (4.5)
Total	**27814**

Table 5.5	Location of procedure and grade of surgeon for NHS day case patients			
Grade of surgeon	**Location of procedure**			
	Theatre suite	Day case unit	Other	Blank
Consultant	8485	6185	465	825
SAS	2339	2235	185	199
SpR 3 and above	1074	586	103	118
SpR 1/2	619	367	59	61
SHO	312	301	46	47
Other	766	970	84	118
Blank	441	572	28	224
Total	**14036**	**11216**	**970**	**1592**

Table 5.6	NHS day case surgery analysed by specialty and grade							
Surgical specialty	**Consultant %**	**SAS %**	**SpR 3 and above %**	**SpR 1/2 %**	**SHO %**	**Other %**	**Blank %**	**Total n=22274**
General	56.5	20.7	5.9	5.8	3.9	5.3	2.0	**3259**
Gynaecology	64.7	15.1	6.3	3.8	1.2	6.0	2.9	**4095**
Ophthalmology	72.6	12.1	8.0	2.7	1.0	1.9	1.7	**5244**
Oral & Maxillofacial	32.3	32.8	3.6	3.6	5.3	18.5	3.9	**1456**
Orthopaedic & Trauma	57.3	23.0	7.8	4.6	0.9	3.7	2.7	**3200**
Otorhino-laryngology	52.9	25.9	5.8	4.7	1.4	6.3	3.1	**1462**
Plastic	31.0	18.2	12.8	9.0	12.2	11.2	5.5	**1176**
Urology	54.2	19.3	7.7	3.6	3.7	8.5	3.1	**2382**

Table 5.5 shows the number of surgeons of each grade caring for day case patients in the NHS divided amongst each location where day patients were treated.

The data were analysed to examine whether some surgical specialties used non-consultant staff more than others.

Table 5.6 shows the proportions of different grades of surgeons, expressed as percentages, that performed day surgery procedures in the surgical specialties that reported more than 1,000 cases.

SHOs operated on 12.2% of plastic surgery patients and 5.3% of oral and maxillofacial surgery patients. In all other surgical specialties the involvement of SHOs was less than 4%. Of the 132 plastic surgery cases where the most senior surgeon present was an SHO, 121 were performed under local anaesthesia, and were mainly excision of skin lesions. The great majority of the cases performed by "Other" surgeons

in oral and maxillofacial surgery were extractions of teeth associated with dental decay under general anaesthesia. These may have been cases that in the past would have been carried out in general dentists' surgeries, until the introduction of the stringent standards that effectively ended general anaesthesia in dentistry outside hospital. In addition, oral and maxillofacial surgery uniquely engages practitioners who hold a dental qualification and who are on a specialist list in surgical dentistry held by the General Dental Council. This means that they are judged competent to practice independently up to a certain level.

ASA STATUS AND GRADE OF DOCTOR

> Trainee doctors were involved in anaesthetising patients of poor health, apparently unsupervised.

Anaesthetics

Table 5.7 shows the number of patients by ASA status who were treated by different grades of anaesthetists, by percentages.

As can be seen, very few of the patients managed as day cases were assessed as ASA 4, 5 or 6. On examination none of the ASA 6 patients were listed as undergoing organ donation, and it is also very likely that the day cases reported as ASA 5 had been wrongly coded. The two ASA 4 patients anaesthetised by SHOs were undergoing cataract extraction under local anaesthesia.

Surgeons

Table 5.8 shows the number of patients of the different ASA grades who were treated by different grades of surgeons, by percentages.

There is a suggestion that patients of ASA 4 were more likely to have a consultant surgeon than patients of ASA 1 to 3, but the numbers assessed at the higher ASA status were small. No operations performed on patients assessed as ASA 4 or 5 were performed by SHOs.

Table 5.7	NHS day case patients analysed by grade of anaesthetist and ASA status							
	ASA status							
Grade of anaesthetist	**1** % n=11405	**2** % n=4873	**3** % n=1060	**4** % n=57	**5** % n=13	**6** % n=18	**Blank** % n=10388	**Total** % n=27814
Consultant	55.2	55.9	60.9	62.7	63.6	40.0	41.0	**50.5**
SAS	16.9	19.4	17.7	15.7	9.1	30.0	13.1	**16.0**
SpR 3 and above	4.0	3.3	3.4	3.9	0.0	0.0	2.4	**3.3**
SpR 1/2	2.8	3.2	2.2	0.0	0.0	10.0	1.5	**2.4**
SHO	3.2	3.2	3.2	3.9	9.1	0.0	1.9	**2.7**
Other	4.6	3.9	3.8	3.9	9.1	0.0	5.9	**4.9**
Blank	13.3	11.1	8.9	9.8	9.1	20.0	34.2	**20.3**

Table 5.8	NHS day case patients analysed by grade of surgeon and ASA grade							
	ASA status							
Grade of surgeon	**1** % n=11405	**2** % n=4873	**3** % n=1060	**4** % n=57	**5** % n=13	**6** % n=18	**Blank** % n=10388	**Total** % n=27814
Consultant	57.7	63.8	63.4	75.4	53.8	27.8	53.4	**57.4**
SAS	18.3	16.6	14.6	7.0	7.7	27.8	18.3	**17.8**
SpR 3 and above	6.8	7.3	7.0	1.8	0.0	27.8	6.5	**6.8**
SpR 1/2	4.1	3.8	3.4	3.5	15.4	11.1	3.9	**4.0**
SHO	2.5	1.4	2.2	0.0	0.0	0.0	3.2	**2.5**
Other	7.6	4.3	4.6	5.3	23.1	<0.1	7.8	**7.0**
Blank	3.1	2.8	4.8	7.0	0.0	5.6	6.9	**4.5**

SUPERVISION OF TRAINEES

> **There was a low level of consultant supervision of trainee anaesthetists.**

Based on the data, day surgery was definitely not a consultant-based service. Consultants gave only 50% of day case anaesthetics and consultants performed 57% of operations. The next biggest staff group was SAS doctors but significant numbers of anaesthetics and operations were being performed when the most senior doctor present was a trainee doctor, including doctors of SHO level. Less experienced doctors were treating not only fit patients but also patients with an ASA status of 3, 4 or 5. This shift away from what has been regarded as good practice in the past is acceptable, so long as there is proper supervision of doctors in training. When dedicated day case units are often sited away from other surgical facilities, it is important that trainees are not left working unsupported in a location geographically distant from more senior help.

When the most senior anaesthetist present was not a consultant, respondents were asked to specify the level of supervision, using the definitions of the Royal College of Anaesthetists. These were:

- Immediately available – in the theatre, or available in the theatre suite without other responsibilities
- Local – on the same geographical site and able to attend within 10 minutes
- Distant – on a different geographical site, or unable to attend within 10 minutes.

Table 5.9 illustrates the level of consultant supervision of trainee anaesthetists working on their own anaesthetising day cases in dedicated day case units.

It is of concern that apparently only one in five SHOs anaesthetising patients on their own was being supervised by a consultant who was immediately available. The numbers may appear small but equate to a total of 5,000 a year.

NCEPOD is unable to judge whether some of the SHOs without immediate consultant supervision might have been able to call on a more senior trainee for assistance. Anaesthetic departments should review their arrangements for the supervision of trainee anaesthetists, especially SHOs, working on their own in dedicated day case units.

Table 5.9	Supervision of trainee anaesthetists				
Level of supervision	Immediately available	Local	Distant	Blank	Total
SpR 3 and above	46	103	78	47	274
SpR 1/2	32	135	19	19	205
SHO	40	75	26	40	181

6 ELECTIVE SURGERY IN THE NHS

INTRODUCTION

Elective operations were those operations to which respondents gave a NCEPOD classification of elective or scheduled. 78% of operations were elective, 15% were non-elective and 8% were not classified.

GRADES OF STAFF FOR ELECTIVE OPERATIONS

Elective surgery was largely performed by career grade staff between the hours of 08.00 and 18.00 on weekdays.

Table 6.1	NHS elective patients by grade of anaesthetist
Grade of anaesthetist	**Number (%) n=49195**
Consultant	26735 (54.3)
SAS	6586 (13.3)
SpR 3 and above	1667 (3.4)
SpR 1/2	1127 (2.3)
SHO	1499 (3.0)
Other	2095 (4.3)
Blank	5400 (11.0)

Table 6.2	NHS elective patients by grade of surgeon
Grade of surgeon	**Number (%) n=49195**
Consultant	31778 (64.6)
SAS	6962 (14.2)
SpR 3 and above	3184 (6.5)
SpR 1/2	1822 (3.7)
SHO	841 (1.7)
Other	2675 (5.4)
Blank	1933 (3.9)

68% of elective patients were anaesthetised by career grade staff where the grade was known to NCEPOD (Table 6.1). 79% of elective patients were operated on by career grade staff (Table 6.2). Less than 6% of cases were treated by the most inexperienced trainees, SHOs, SpR 1s and SpR 2s working unsupervised.

THE TYPE OF SESSION USED FOR ELECTIVE OPERATIONS

Most hospitals have followed previous NCEPOD recommendations and have theatre sessions planned for emergency surgery, and also scheduled sessions for trauma. It has been suggested that these sessions are misused, and that elective patients have been operated on in NCEPOD theatres or in emergency theatres out of hours. The types of theatre session used for elective surgery have been analysed (Table 6.3).

Only 795 elective cases were done on scheduled emergency lists (out of a total of 49,195 classified as elective – 1.7%). A further 244 (0.5%) were done in unscheduled time. This would appear to suggest that NCEPOD lists were not grossly abused.

These data can also be analysed to see the proportions of elective and non-elective cases carried out on NCEPOD lists (Table 6.4).

A modest number of elective cases were performed on NCEPOD lists and in unscheduled sessions.

Trusts should monitor the use of NCEPOD lists. They should ensure that urgent and emergency cases are not delayed because these lists are being used for elective cases.

The number of Trusts that have NCEPOD lists and the pressures on such lists are considered further in Chapter 7.

Table 6.3	NHS elective cases by type of theatre session by day of week				
	Scheduled (%) n=47789	Emergency surgical (%) n=361	Emergency trauma (%) n=434	Unscheduled (%) n=244	Blank (%) n=367
Monday	9665 (20.2)	44 (12.2)	72 (16.6)	18 (7.4)	58 (15.8)
Tuesday	9137 (19.1)	69 (19.1)	65 (15.0)	39 (16.0)	68 (18.5)
Wednesday	9435 (19.7)	57 (15.8)	82 (18.9)	23 (9.4)	73 (19.9)
Thursday	9292 (19.4)	70 (19.4)	69 (15.9)	38 (15.6)	66 (18.0)
Friday	8098 (16.9)	68 (18.8)	84 (19.4)	36 (14.8)	71 (19.3)
Saturday	1753 (3.7)	29 (8.0)	41 (9.4)	68 (27.9)	22 (6.0)
Sunday	305 (0.6)	23 (6.4)	19 (4.4)	22 (9.0)	3 (0.8)
Blank	104 (0.2)	1 (0.3)	2 (0.5)	0 (0.0)	6 (1.6)

Table 6.4	Elective and non-elective cases by type of theatre session				
Type of case	Scheduled (%) n=52770	Emergency surgical (%) n=5082	Emergency trauma (%) n=3236	Unscheduled (%) n=1181	Blank (%) n=1240
Elective	47789 (91)	361 (7)	434 (13)	244 (21)	367 (30)
Non-elective	1401 (3)	4324 (85)	2503 (77)	859 (73)	123 (10)
Blank	3580 (7)	397 (8)	299 (9)	78 (7)	750 (60)

WHEN WERE ELECTIVE CASES DONE?

4.5% of elective operations were performed at the weekend.

There have been moves to extend the working day by performing elective surgery in the evenings and weekends (Table 6.5).

Only a small amount of elective surgery appears to have been done in the evening, but a substantial number of cases were reported as being done at the weekend. These are likely to be additional cases done under various waiting list initiatives. (The 25 cases reported as having operations at the weekend under the care of an Accident & Emergency consultant were all minor body surface operations at the same hospital.)

If elective cases are done outside the normal working day it is important that the patients' physical statuses are appropriate, that the correct grade of staff are present for the operations, and that the facilities are equivalent to those available during the day.

Selection of cases

ASA status was used as a surrogate marker for the physical status of the patient. Table 6.6 gives the numbers of elective patients, expressed as counts and then as percentages, of each ASA status for different times of the week.

There does not appear to be any tendency for patients of better (or worse) ASA status to have been operated on at a particular time of day. Of the 29 elective ASA 3 patients whose anaesthetic or operation started between 00.00 and 07.59, 24 were undergoing cardiac surgery, probably as the first patient on a daytime list.

Table 6.5	Times of NHS elective operations by specialty						
Specialty of surgeon	**Weekday 08:00 to 17:59**	**Weekday 18:00 to 23:59**	**Weekend 08:00 to 17:59**	**Weekend 18:00 to 23:59**	**Night 00:00 to 07:59**	**Blank**	**% of cases weekend 08:00 to 17:59**
Accident and Emergency	37	2	25	0	0	1	38.5
Cardiac/Thoracic/Cardiothoracic	733	6	30	0	29	4	3.7
General	6935	53	387	4	7	84	5.2
Gynaecology	5880	23	180	2	2	85	2.9
Neurosurgery	369	3	8	0	0	10	2.1
Ophthalmology	5512	77	337	2	3	53	5.6
Oral & Maxillofacial	1807	4	47	0	2	39	2.5
Orthopaedic & Trauma	6937	68	426	10	21	85	5.6
Other	980	11	43	1	1	18	4.1
Otorhinolaryngology	3910	23	204	2	3	67	4.8
Paediatrics	541	4	7	0	0	6	1.3
Plastic	1692	28	93	5	4	19	5.1
Transplantation	65	0	0	0	0	1	<0.1
Urology	4261	14	133	0	9	76	3.0
Vascular	902	6	42	2	0	10	4.4
Blank	5111	52	241	2	5	272	4.2
Total	**45672**	**374**	**2203**	**30**	**86**	**830**	**4.5**

Table 6.6	Analysis of NHS elective patients by time and ASA status					
ASA status	**Weekday 08:00 to 17:59**	**Weekday 18:00 to 23:59**	**Weekend 08:00 to 17:59**	**Weekend 18:00 to 23:59**	**Night 00:00 to 07:59**	**Blank**
1	16288	146	763	12	16	212
2	10471	88	457	5	19	84
3	3868	29	158	4	29	18
4	375	1	15	0	0	4
5	28	0	2	0	0	0
6	17	0	0	0	0	0
Blank	14625	110	808	9	22	512
Total	**45672**	**374**	**2203**	**30**	**86**	**830**

THE GRADES OF ANAESTHETIST AND SURGEON

Consultant anaesthetists and surgeons were the most senior clinician present for two-thirds of cases at weekends.

Anaesthetists

Table 6.7 shows the number of elective patients by the grade of the most senior anaesthetist present at different times of the week.

During the normal working day, weekdays 08.00 to 17.59, consultants anaesthetised 60% of patients. The anaesthetist was more often a consultant during the daytime at weekends – 69% of cases. On review of the six cases done at a weekend between 18.00 and 23.59, where the most senior anaesthetist present was a consultant, it is probable that most were non-elective cases that had been incorrectly reported as elective.

Surgeons

Table 6.8 shows the number of elective patients by the grade of the most senior surgeon present at different times of the week.

A consultant was the surgeon in two-thirds of cases during the daytime, both during the week and at weekends. The high figure of 77% for the involvement of a consultant surgeon at night reflects that most of those were early starts of elective cardiac operations. As noted above, the cases performed between 18.00 and 23.59 at weekends appear to be incorrectly classified non-elective operations of a relatively minor complexity.

Table 6.7	Analysis of NHS elective patients by time and grade of anaesthetist					
Grade of anaesthetist	Weekday 08:00 to 17:59	Weekday 18:00 to 23:59	Weekend 08:00 to 17:59	Weekend 18:00 to 23:59	Night 00:00 to 07:59	Blank
Consultant	24820	189	1363	6	61	296
SAS	6158	32	324	3	7	62
SpR 3 and above	1621	8	20	5	1	12
SpR 1/2	1104	4	6	3	1	9
SHO	1414	30	32	11	2	10
Other	2003	16	42	0	0	34
Blank	4807	49	201	2	13	328
Total	**41927**	**328**	**1988**	**30**	**85**	**751**

Table 6.8	Analysis of NHS elective patients by time and grade of surgeon					
Grade of surgeon	Weekday 08:00 to 17:59	Weekday 18:00 to 23:59	Weekend 08:00 to 17:59	Weekend 18:00 to 23:59	Night 00:00 to 07:59	Blank
Consultant	29664	222	1421	9	66	396
SAS	6327	73	450	2	10	100
SpR 3 and above	3008	23	104	2	2	45
SpR 1/2	1715	14	56	11	3	23
SHO	812	5	5	1	1	17
Other	2496	22	89	5	1	62
Blank	1650	15	78	0	3	187
Total	**45672**	**374**	**2203**	**30**	**86**	**830**

RECOVERY FACILITIES

It is important that all the facilities necessary are available for elective operating outside the normal working day, not just the operating theatre, theatre personnel and doctors.

Respondents were asked, *"Would the arrangements for the recovery of this patient prevent the start of another case (if required)?"* (Table 6.9).

Recovery facilities appear to have been properly organised for elective cases, whether done during normal hours or as part of an extended day in the evening or at the weekend, apart from the increased number of delays for the relatively small number of operations carried out on weekday evenings.

For elective operating outside traditional working hours, the overall picture is reassuring. The seniority of anaesthetists and surgeons was similar to that during weekday daytimes. Work at unsociable hours was not being delegated to SAS doctors or trainees. The numbers of staff available to recover patients appear to have been adequate and the ASA statuses of the patients were not significantly different than during normal working hours. This report cannot comment on whether the staff available to recover patients, had at all times, been properly trained in this role, nor whether the facilities elsewhere in the hospital were provided to an appropriate standard.

Table 6.9	Recovery arrangements for elective NHS patients at different times of the week					
Start of next case prevented	Weekday 08:00 to 17:59 (%) n=45672	Weekday 18:00 to 23:59 (%) n=374	Weekend 08:00 to 17:59 (%) n=2203	Weekend 18:00 to 23:59 (%) n=30	Night 00:00 to 07:59 (%) n=86	Blank (%) n=830
Yes	1490 (3.3)	26 (7.0)	53 (2.4)	5 (16.7)	5 (5.8)	20 (2.4)
No	37850 (82.9)	278 (74.3)	1779 (80.8)	17 (56.7)	59 (68.6)	567 (68.3)
Blank	6332 (13.9)	70 (18.7)	371 (16.8)	8 (26.7)	22 (25.6)	243 (29.3)

Recommendations

Debate whether, in the light of changes to the pattern of junior doctors' working, non-essential surgery can take place during extended hours.

Ensure that all essential services (including emergency operating rooms, recovery rooms, high dependency units and intensive care units) are provided on a single site wherever emergency/acute surgical care is delivered.

7 NON-ELECTIVE SURGERY IN THE NHS

INTRODUCTION

Non-elective operations are those which meet the NCEPOD criteria as either:

"Emergency", operation simultaneously with resuscitation, usually within one hour, or:

"Urgent", operation as soon as possible after resuscitation, usually within 24 hours.

Non-elective operations made up nearly 16% of the surgical workload in NHS hospitals.

WHICH SPECIALTIES ARE INVOLVED IN NON-ELECTIVE WORK?

There were large differences between specialties in the proportion of the total specialty workload made up of non-elective cases.

Table 7.1 — Breakdown by specialty and classification

Surgical specialty	Elective	Non-elective	Non-elective %	Total
Accident and Emergency	65	10	13.3	75
Cardiac/Thoracic/Cardiothoracic	802	165	17.1	967
General	7470	2008	21.2	9478
Gynaecology	6172	921	13.0	7093
Neurosurgery	390	165	29.7	555
Ophthalmology	5984	165	2.7	6149
Oral & Maxillofacial	1899	179	8.6	2078
Orthopaedic & Trauma	7547	2632	25.9	10179
Otorhinolaryngology	4209	221	5.0	4430
Paediatrics	558	191	25.5	749
Plastic	1841	627	25.4	2468
Transplantation	66	25	27.5	91
Urology	4493	188	4.0	4681
Vascular	962	291	23.2	1253
Other	1054	148	12.3	1202
Blank	5683	1274	18.3	6957
Total	**49195**	**9210**	**15.8**	**58405**

Table 7.2 — Time of non-elective NHS operations by specialty

Specialty of surgeon	Weekday 08:00 to 17:59		Weekday 18:00 to 23:59		Weekend 08:00 to 17:59		Weekend 18:00 to 23:59		Night 00:00 to 07:59		Blank		Total	
Accident and Emergency	7	0.1%	0	0.0%	2	<0.1%	1	<0.1%	0	0.0%	0	0.0%	10	0.1%
Cardiac/Thoracic/Cardiothoracic	120	1.3%	21	0.2%	13	0.1%	2	<0.1%	9	0.1%	0	0.0%	165	1.8%
General	867	9.4%	561	6.1%	300	3.3%	139	1.5%	121	1.3%	20	0.2%	2008	21.8%
Gynaecology/Obstetrics	533	5.8%	207	2.2%	96	1.0%	31	0.3%	41	0.4%	13	0.1%	921	10.0%
Neurosurgery	81	0.9%	35	0.4%	24	0.3%	9	0.1%	15	0.2%	1	<0.1%	165	1.8%
Ophthalmology	124	1.3%	18	0.2%	16	0.2%	1	<0.1%	4	<0.1%	2	<0.1%	165	1.8%
Oral & Maxillofacial	102	1.1%	23	0.2%	38	0.4%	10	0.1%	3	0.0%	3	<0.1%	179	1.9%
Orthopaedic & Trauma	1400	15.2%	374	4.1%	610	6.6%	155	1.7%	55	0.6%	38	0.4%	2632	28.6%
Other	75	0.8%	31	0.3%	26	0.3%	10	0.1%	4	<0.1%	2	<0.1%	148	1.6%
Otorhinolaryngology	139	1.5%	27	0.3%	27	0.3%	15	0.2%	12	0.1%	1	<0.1%	221	2.4%
Paediatrics	106	1.2%	42	0.5%	26	0.3%	7	0.1%	10	0.1%	0	0.0%	191	2.1%
Plastic	321	3.5%	122	1.3%	137	1.5%	37	0.4%	4	<0.1%	6	0.1%	627	6.8%
Transplantation	12	0.1%	5	0.1%	8	0.1%	0	0.0%	0	0.0%	0	0.0%	25	0.3%
Urology	118	1.3%	28	0.3%	23	0.2%	11	0.1%	5	0.1%	3	<0.1%	188	2.0%
Vascular	162	1.8%	68	0.7%	30	0.3%	14	0.2%	16	0.2%	1	<0.1%	291	3.2%
Blank	689	7.5%	233	2.5%	177	1.9%	76	0.8%	49	0.5%	50	0.5%	1274	13.8%
Total	**4856**	**52.7%**	**1795**	**19.5%**	**1553**	**16.9%**	**518**	**5.6%**	**348**	**3.8%**	**140**	**1.5%**	**9210**	**100.0%**

Table 7.1 illustrates the elective and non-elective work for surgical specialties. NHS cases where no classification of the theatre case was given, totalled 5,104/63,509.

Overall, 15.8% of the total workload were non-elective cases. This figure disguises considerable variation between specialties. Ophthalmology, otorhinolaryngology and urology had large numbers of cases, but very few were non-elective. Other specialties had much larger numbers of non-elective cases forming a significant part of their workload. Obviously different specialties will require different strategies to manage their elective workload whilst ensuring that non-elective cases are treated promptly.

Table 7.2 details when non-elective operations took place throughout the week. Just over 50% of cases were done during normal working hours.

Specialties carry out non-elective operations at different times. Figure 7.1 analyses the times when surgery was done in the four specialties with the biggest non-elective workload.

Gynaecology patients were most likely to have their operations during the week, whilst orthopaedic and trauma and plastic surgery had a bigger proportion of their non-elective workload at weekends. General surgery performed the smallest proportion of non-elective cases in the daytime during the week.

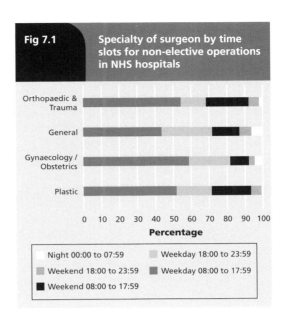

Fig 7.1 Specialty of surgeon by time slots for non-elective operations in NHS hospitals

Legend:
- Night 00:00 to 07:59
- Weekday 18:00 to 23:59
- Weekend 18:00 to 23:59
- Weekday 08:00 to 17:59
- Weekend 08:00 to 17:59

The impact on hospitals

The data can also be used to examine which specialties contribute to the total non-elective workload (Figure 7.2).

This chart shows all the data reported to NCEPOD. The proportions relating to the common specialties are probably applicable to most hospitals. Only tertiary hospitals will have carried out non-elective operations in such specialties as neurosurgery and cardiothoracic surgery. These specialties may have had a significant impact on the overall pattern of non-elective work in their hospitals.

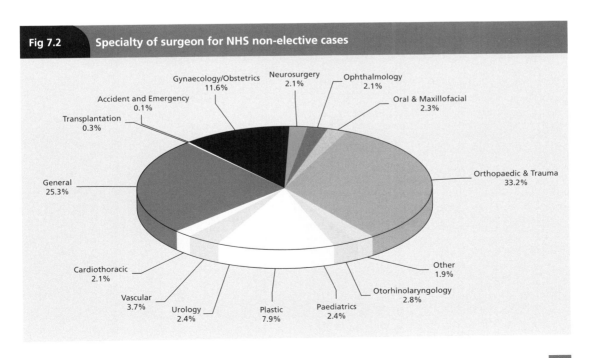

Fig 7.2 Specialty of surgeon for NHS non-elective cases

- Gynaecology/Obstetrics 11.6%
- Neurosurgery 2.1%
- Ophthalmology 2.1%
- Oral & Maxillofacial 2.3%
- Accident and Emergency 0.1%
- Transplantation 0.3%
- Orthopaedic & Trauma 33.2%
- General 25.3%
- Other 1.9%
- Cardiothoracic 2.1%
- Otorhinolaryngology 2.8%
- Vascular 3.7%
- Urology 2.4%
- Plastic 7.9%
- Paediatrics 2.4%

USE OF NCEPOD LISTS

The 1990 NCEPOD report [7] recommended the provision of dedicated emergency operating theatres. Table 7.3 shows how many non-elective cases were done on planned emergency operating lists.

162 hospitals out of 395 that responded reported that they provided scheduled daytime staffed lists for trauma patients, and 171 out of 395 hospitals ran scheduled daytime staffed lists for general emergencies. Trusts may manage more than one hospital, with only one hospital in the Trust having scheduled emergency lists. Data returned to NCEPOD for the 2001 report [20] showed that in a random sample of 1,467 patients who died within 30 days of surgery, 86% had been treated in a hospital with daytime trauma lists and 78% had been treated in a hospital with daytime lists for general emergencies.

During the week, the majority of daytime non-elective operations were done in sessions scheduled for emergency operating. The number of operations at weekends reported as being done in scheduled emergency sessions is surprisingly high.

Between 08.00 and 17.59 on weekdays, 26% (1,269/4,856) of non-elective cases were done on scheduled lists (Table 7.3). There are at least two possible explanations for this. Some elective lists are planned to have enough spare capacity for non-elective cases to be added as necessary. Secondly, if elective patients planned for an elective list have to be cancelled (for example, because of a shortage of available beds in the hospital) then the time can be used for patients waiting for non-elective surgery.

Consultant surgeon:

"...if you don't get your elective admissions in, you can often do emergency cases on those lists...it ameliorates our emergency surgery problems considerably."

One of the earliest recommendations of NCEPOD was that "Essential services (including emergency operating rooms, recovery rooms, high dependency units and intensive care units) must be provided on a single site wherever emergency/acute surgical care is delivered" [7]. It is worth rehearsing the reasons why this recommendation is still valid.

If emergency operating theatres are not made available, all the operating theatres in a hospital will be allocated during the day to elective work. An elective list might be interrupted for an emergency case, but the great majority of non-elective cases would wait until the evening when elective operating had finished. This policy is unsatisfactory. Firstly, it shows no consideration for the mental state of the patient, or the pain and discomfort suffered whilst waiting for surgery. Secondly, the physical condition of the patient might deteriorate because of the delay. Thirdly, there is usually a queue of patients waiting for surgery when a theatre does become available at 18.00, so that inevitably operations that could have been done in daylight hours start well into the evening or even after midnight. Finally, operations that are urgent, but not emergencies, that might be able to wait until morning, will be done at night because the staff know that a wait until the morning of the next day actually means a wait until the evening of the next day.

These concerns are compounded by the problems associated with anaesthesia and surgery out of hours.

Theatre staff at night may be less experienced in certain surgical specialties or in using sophisticated

Table 7.3	Breakdown of NHS non-elective cases by session type					
	Scheduled	**Emergency surgical**	**Emergency trauma**	**Unscheduled**	**Blank**	**Total**
Monday to Friday 08:00 - 17:59	1269	1927	1316	248	96	4856
Monday to Friday 18:00 - 07:59	35	1289	403	315	5	2047
Saturday to Sunday 00:00 - 23:59	81	1065	741	292	16	2195
Blank	16	43	43	4	6	112
Total	**1401**	**4324**	**2503**	**859**	**123**	**9210**

equipment. Some specialised surgery may require teams to be brought in from home, delaying the start of non-elective cases and possibly compromising elective work next day. There are fewer staff in the rest of the hospital, such as radiographers, ward nursing staff, laboratory staff and porters, and this may reduce the quality of care and cause delays. Work is more likely to be performed by trainee doctors who at times have underestimated the severity of a patient's condition and undertaken work beyond their competence.

The institution of daytime lists for emergency operating has been a major improvement in the quality of care delivered to surgical patients. The role of this enquiry in bringing about this change is reflected in the name usually given to these facilities, NCEPOD lists or NCEPOD theatres. Unfortunately the provision of these emergency operating theatres is still subject to problems.

As shown in Chapter 8 as to why operations were done out of hours, some hospitals still do not have emergency operating theatres at all; one consultant commented:

"We do not have an emergency gynaecology theatre."

and another,

"This 22 year-old patient … waited over 30 hours for appendicectomy due to unavailability of theatre space during daytime working hours."

Staffing an emergency theatre continues to be problematic. When an emergency theatre is established, resources are usually made available for theatre staff, and there will often an anaesthetist allocated to emergency duties.

It has been more difficult to ensure that surgical staff are available to operate in NCEPOD theatres during the day. Figures given above show that the non-elective workload varies considerably between specialties. Trauma theatres work well for orthopaedic urgent cases. In some hospitals, consultants in general surgery are now released from elective work to concentrate on non-elective work.

It is recognised that for smaller specialties such as paediatric surgery and maxillofacial surgery it is more difficult to have senior staff available for non-elective work because there are fewer surgeons and the emergency workload is less. This is shown by the replies in Chapter 8 detailing "Surgeon of the correct grade not available".

Hospitals may have established NCEPOD theatres, but if they serve a large population and have a heavy emergency load, this capacity may not be enough to ensure that no non-elective cases that could be done in daylight hours are left to be done out of hours. Many respondents reported that there was too much emergency work in their hospitals to be done in the NCEPOD operating time available.

"There are inevitable delays on these emergency operating lists and sometimes patients with hand injuries wait a good number of hours. The problem would be solved with a plastic trauma list." (reply to an out of hours questionnaire)

Another problem for emergency operating sessions is that emergency work is not given the same priority as elective work.

"Although a separate CEPOD (sic) theatre is available during most days of the week, the political situation means that often in practice the elective lists take precedence over the CEPOD (sic) theatre. On the day in question only two small cases were done during the day." (reply to an out of hours questionnaire)

The Audit Commission recently reviewed the efficient use of scheduled theatre time [2]. Based on their findings that scheduled general emergency operating sessions were used for between 38 and 63% of the allocated time it specified an arbitrary target of 60% utilisation for these sessions. The caption to one exhibit in the Audit Commission report states, "Trusts above the 60% utilisation line have too many scheduled sessions". This comment was picked up in a British Medical Journal news item [21], which reported it as "To get more out of each theatre, hospitals could reduce the number of sessions they leave clear for emergencies". This was misleading because the Audit Commission report then examined why scheduled emergency sessions might be underused, echoing the factors listed above. If sufficient facilities are provided so that most patients will not have undue waits for treatment, then there will be occasions when the facilities will not be used.

The information collected by NCEPOD indicates that scheduled emergency operating sessions are essential for good patient care, and that Trusts should address the obstacles to the proper use of these facilities. Patients admitted as emergencies deserve as much consideration as elective patients admitted from waiting lists.

WHO OPERATES ON NON-ELECTIVE CASES?

> The involvement of senior staff has markedly increased since WOW I.

Anaesthetics

Table 7.4 shows each grade by time period, for non-elective NHS patients. The corresponding figures for WOW I have been included for comparison. The figures for the different grades that were collected for this report have been combined, so that the grades in the figures for "SpR 3 and above" approximate to a senior registrar in WOW I, and the grades "SpR 1/2" approximate to a registrar.

Consultants and SAS doctors were much more involved than in 1995/96, at all times of the day and night. This is commendable. Comment was made in WOW I that whilst routine (elective) cases were mainly done by consultants or other experienced staff, emergency (non-elective) work was the province of the trainee. There has been a definite change in the anaesthetic management of non-elective work but the tradition continues for out of hours cover to be provided mainly by trainees.

Surgery

Table 7.5 shows the numbers for each grade of surgeon as percentages of the total for each time period, again compared to WOW I.

Again, "SpR 3 and above" approximates to the grade of senior registrar in WOW I, and "SpR 1/2" to registrar.

Surgical consultants, and SAS doctors, were much more involved than in 1995/96, at all times of the day and night. This is again commendable. Comparing the figures from WOW I and WOW II, the reduction in the proportion of non-elective work done by SpR 1/2 doctors is remarkable.

A number of factors have to be taken into account when deciding how best to allocate non-elective

Table 7.4	Grade of anaesthetist by time of day compared to WOW I					
Grade of anaesthetist	**Day**		**Evening**		**Night**	
	WOW I	**WOW II**	**WOW I**	**WOW II**	**WOW I**	**WOW II**
Consultant	26.2%	44.5%	9.4%	17.6%	9.0%	18.0%
SAS	7.4%	12.7%	4.8%	8.9%	4.6%	6.1%
SpR 3 and above	7.7%	7.3%	8.8%	12.4%	12.2%	13.4%
SpR 1/2	15.9%	4.7%	19.3%	7.3%	23.3%	9.0%
SHO	35.3%	18.5%	51.5%	38.2%	44.3%	36.9%
Other	5.2%	6.2%	3.8%	9.8%	4.0%	9.6%
Blank	2.2%	6.0%	2.3%	5.7%	2.7%	7.0%
Total	**4645**	**6425**	**2871**	**2320**	**524**	**348**

Table 7.5	Grade of surgeon by time of day compared to WOW I					
Grade of surgeon	**Day**		**Evening**		**Night**	
	WOW I	**WOW II**	**WOW I**	**WOW II**	**WOW I**	**WOW II**
Consultant	28.5%	41.4%	14.2%	20.6%	11.4%	25.6%
SAS	7.3%	14.5%	5.9%	16.1%	5.6%	11.5%
SpR 3 and above	13.3%	14.1%	13.1%	19.4%	15.0%	22.1%
SpR 1/2	33.0%	11.0%	41.5%	13.9%	42.9%	13.5%
SHO	13.4%	5.0%	21.9%	9.0%	22.3%	6.6%
Other	2.1%	9.2%	1.3%	14.7%	0.9%	12.6%
Blank	2.4%	4.8%	2.1%	6.3%	1.9%	8.0%
Total	**4993**	**6425**	**2986**	**2320**	**534**	**348**

work between different grades of staff. Non-elective cases have the potential to be very challenging. The patient may be very sick, both because of their presenting condition and because of co-morbidities, yet there may be limited time available to improve the patient's condition. In such circumstances it is essential that senior staff are involved, to decide the optimal time for surgery and to perform the actual anaesthesia and surgery. On the other hand, many non-elective patients are fit and require simple surgery, so that the case may be within the competence of relatively inexperienced trainees. Trainees need to spend time working independently as part of their training, but such opportunities are becoming less common. In the right setting, simple non-elective cases done by trainees working on their own, with appropriate supervision available, can be an important and appropriate part of their training, without detriment to the patient.

One of the reasons for restricting non-essential operating at night is that doctors working on-call rotas would be tired having worked all day. It has been suggested that trainee doctors should be doing more cases at night now that their hours are protected. Because of the new working patterns, trainees will be fresh when coming on duty in the evening, and they will not be expected to be involved in patient care the next day if they have been working during the night.

The advisors expressed concerns about how this would be implemented in practice. Hospitals effectively shut down at night, so that the resources of ward staff, radiology and laboratory staff would not be able to support a significant extra operating at night. Of particular concern is how consultant supervision is going to be provided without shift working and a dramatic increase in the number of consultants. The issues should be debated as a matter of urgency by Royal Colleges, professional bodies, DoH and the British Medical Association (BMA) amongst others.

8 INVESTIGATION OF OUT OF HOURS CASES IN THE NHS

INTRODUCTION

A letter was sent to the consultant anaesthetist and the consultant surgeon in charge of each case that was identified as having taken place out of hours. The letter asked for information as to why the case had been done at that time.

THE REASONS FOR OUT OF HOURS SURGERY

> **Many consultants do not regard their work outside the hours 08.00 to 18.00 as "out of hours".**

This exercise mirrored a similar exercise in WOW I, when a letter was sent to the surgeon only. The intention was to understand whether a case was done out of hours as part of planned elective activity, because of pressing clinical need for a non-elective case, or whether with better planning and resources, the case could have been done within normal working hours.

"Out of hours" was defined for this report as any time outside 08.00 to 17.59 on weekdays, and any time on a Saturday or Sunday. This is the same definition that was used in WOW I. Some respondents felt this definition was too restrictive.

"Normal working hours in the NHS … is up to 21.00 for anaesthetic consultants."

"17.00 on a Saturday, not out of hours."

"13.00 on a Sunday is not out of hours."

There were several comments in this vein. These replies, together with the other data in the report, show that consultants spend considerable amounts of time in NHS hospitals outside the traditional standard working day of 9 to 5 on weekdays.

Most respondents were helpful.

"In reply to your letter, firstly my apologies for the delay in getting this back to you but I have only just obtained the hospital records."

Some were upset by the request for information and obviously misunderstood the purpose of the exercise.

"I think it is outrageous that you are asking me to justify best practice for operating out of hours. Had I not operated on this case I would have been sued for negligence. We are overwhelmed with bureaucracy and this is just adding to the burden."

> **Many operations were performed out of hours because of inadequate scheduled sessions for non-elective surgery.**

The replies received were reviewed by NCEPOD clinical co-ordinators, and allocated into appropriate categories (Tables 8.1 and 8.2).

Table 8.1	Anaesthetists' replies	
Anaesthetic out of hours reason	**Count** n=2481	**(%)**
Justified on clinical grounds	1756	(70.8)
Daytime emergency theatre already fully utilised	144	(5.8)
No daytime emergency theatre	108	(4.4)
Evening/weekend trauma list	97	(3.9)
Did not need to be done out of hours	55	(2.2)
Surgeon of the correct grade not available	32	(1.3)
Surgeon requested a time out of hours	21	(0.8)
Waiting list initiative	13	(0.5)
Wait for patient to be starved	12	(0.5)
Elective list over run	11	(0.4)
Other	8	(0.3)
No information supplied	224	(9.0)

Table 8.2	Surgeons' replies	
Surgical out of hours reason	**Count** n=2597	**(%)**
Justified on clinical grounds	1706	(65.7)
Daytime emergency theatre already fully utilised	275	(10.6)
No daytime emergency theatre	163	(6.3)
Evening/weekend trauma list	121	(4.7)
Did not need to be done out of hours	107	(4.1)
Surgeon of the correct grade not available	10	(0.4)
Surgeon requested a time out of hours	9	(0.3)
Waiting list initiative	6	(0.2)
Wait for patient to be starved	6	(0.2)
Elective list over run	11	(0.4)
Other	5	(0.2)
No information supplied	178	(6.9)

The replies from anaesthetists and surgeons cannot be compared directly because in some cases a reply was received from the consultant anaesthetist but not the consultant surgeon, and in other cases *vice versa*. Overall the two samples are consistent, with the clinical co-ordinators considering that in approximately two thirds of the cases the replies justified the decision to perform the operation out of hours on clinical grounds. In 2% of the anaesthetists' replies, and 4% of the surgeons' replies, there appeared to be no justification for carrying out the operation outside normal hours.

In 10% of the anaesthetists' replies, and 17% of the surgeons', the case could have been done during normal working hours if there had been sufficient scheduled lists for emergency operating.

In some cases the hospital did not have any scheduled emergency lists for general emergencies or for trauma (NCEPOD lists), at all. Most hospitals have had NCEPOD lists in some form for many years. Their doctors and managers have begun to devote a just and sensible share of resources to the proper care of emergency cases, to the benefit of those patients. It is hard to understand why some Trusts have failed to follow their lead.

In others, the hospital did have such lists but the case in question still had to be done out of hours. In some cases this may have been because the list had been used inefficiently, but there are undoubtedly large hospitals, which have such an amount of non-elective work from all surgical specialties that they can justify scheduling more sessions for non-orthopaedic emergency operating than they do at the moment.

NCEPOD lists are considered further in the chapter on non-elective surgery.

NIGHT TIME CASES

At first sight these Tables 8.3 to 8.14 appear to include a significant number of cases normally considered elective but performed at night. Further analysis reveals that many of these cases are in fact started early in the morning on an elective list.

(The figures in brackets appear to be true 'night time' surgery as opposed to elective lists starting early). Where possible we have tried to highlight this but it may not be 100% accurate owing to the fact that NCEPOD are not aware of the exact times that hospitals start elective lists. In fact it is known that different specialties within the same hospital will start their lists at different times.

81 cases were omitted due to missing procedure or specialty of surgeon.

Table 8.3	Cardiothoracic		
Classification of case	**Procedure**	**Count**	
Emergency	Re-opening of chest for bleeding	2	(2)
	Coronary artery bypass graft(s)	1	(1)
	Bronchoscopy & removal of tissue from stent	1	(1)
	Re-opening of chest for re-grafting	1	(1)
	Heart transplant	1	(1)
	Post-operative cardiac bleeding	1	(1)
Urgent	Drainage of pericardial effusion	1	(1)
Scheduled	Coronary artery bypass graft(s)	11	
	Aortic valve replacement	5	
	Replacement of right ventricular outflow conduit	1	
Elective	Coronary artery bypass graft(s)	8	
	Mitral valve replacement	1	
	Aortic valve replacement	2	
	Mitral & aortic valve replacement	1	
	Repair of thoracic aortic aneurysm	1	
Blank	Coronary artery bypass graft(s)	2	
	Re-opening of sternum	1	

Table 8.4	Otorhinolaryngology		
Classification of case	**Procedure**	**Count**	
Emergency	Control of primary post tonsillectomy haemorrhage	4	(4)
	Exploration of neck and securing haemostasis & flap from chest wall	1	(1)
	F.E.S.S.	1	
	Intubation for supraglottitis	1	(1)
Urgent	External ethmoidectomy inferior antrostomy	1	
	Removal of fishbone from oesophagus	1	(1)
	Foreign body removal	2	(2)
Scheduled	Adenotonsillectomy	1	
	Bilateral functional endoscopic sinus surgery	1	(1)
Blank	Oesophagoscopy for removal of coin	1	(1)
	Bronchoscopy and intubation	1	(1)

Table 8.5	Maxillofacial		
Classification of case	**Procedure**	**Count**	
Emergency	Tracheostomy and incision & drainage submandibular abcess	1	(1)
Urgent	Repeat venous anastomosis end to side IJV to cephalic vein	1	(1)
Elective	Neck dissection	2	

Table 8.6 — Neurosurgery

Classification of case	Procedure	Count	
Emergency	External ventricular drain	3	(3)
	Cranitomy & evacuation of haematoma	2	(2)
	Burr holes	2	(2)
	Evacuation extradural haematoma	1	(1)
	Revision of VP shunt	1	(1)
	Evacuation extradural & subdural heamatoma	1	(1)
	Burr hole and insertion of ventricular drain	1	(1)
	Elevation of depressed skull fracture	1	(1)
Urgent	Craniotomy	1	(1)
	Removal of VP shunt & insertion of external ventricular drain	1	(1)
Blank	Craniotomy	1	(1)

Table 8.7 — Ophthalmology

Classification of case	Procedure	Count	
Emergency	Vitreous tap intraviteous antibiotics	1	
	Corneal graft	1	(1)
Urgent	Injection of drug into vitreous, biopsy of vitreous	1	(1)
	Right upper lid sutured	1	(1)
Scheduled	Cataract	1	
Elective	Phako + IOL	1	

Table 8.8 — Paediatric surgery

Classification of case	Procedure	Count	
Emergency	Transplantation of liver	1	
	Laparotomy and resection of bowel	1	(1)
	Exploration of left hemiscrotum	1	(1)
	Appendicectomy	1	(1)
	Bladder ultrasound insertion urethral catheter and bladder irrigation	1	(1)
	Laparotomy and ileal resection for intussception	1	(1)
	Left orchidectomy & right orchidopexy	1	(1)
Urgent	Exploration of scar	1	(1)
	Laparotomy and ileostomy	1	(1)
	Suture of vulva	1	(1)
Blank	Testicular exploration and fixation	1	(1)

Table 8.9 — Plastic surgery

Classification of case	Procedure	Count	
Emergency	Revision of skin flap, harvest of veins, evacuation of haematoma	1	(1)
	Incision drainage washout of laceration to finger	1	(1)
	Resection of brachial artery & basilic vein graft	1	(1)
Urgent	Aspiration of haematoma	1	(1)
Scheduled	Abdominoplasty	1	(1)
Elective	Removal K wire inter bone fixation	1	

Table 8.10 — Urology

Classification of case	Procedure	Count	
Emergency	Fixation for testicular torsion	1	(1)
	Exploration of testis and ligation of patent processus vaginalis-groin approach	1	(1)
	Drainage of scrotum	1	(1)
Urgent	Fixation of testis	1	(1)
	Debridement skin – necrotic scrotum	1	(1)
Scheduled	EUA & Cystoscopy	1	
	Bilateral hydrocele	1	

Table 8.11 **General**

Classification of case	Procedure	Count	
Emergency	Laparotomy	12	(12)
	Liver transplant	1	
	Inguinal herniotomy	1	(1)
	Haemorrhage - post haemorrhoidectomy	1	
	Double-barrelled stoma	1	(1)
	Exploration of scrotum	2	(2)
	Exploration of testicles	2	(2)
	Exploration of groin	2	(2)
	Laparoscopy	1	(1)
	Femoral embolectomy	1	(1)
	AAA repair	3	(3)
	Hartmann's	2	(2)
	Lymph node excision	1	(1)
	Gastroscopy	1	(1)
	Laparotomy & splenectomy	2	(2)
	Femoral hernia repair	2	(2)
	Repair of bleeding duodenal ulcer	4	(4)
	Exploration of multiple stab wounds	1	(1)
	Endoscopy	1	(1)
	Laparotomy & insertion of sengstaken tube	1	(1)
	Subtotal colectomy and ileostomy	1	(1)
	Evacuation of haematoma	1	(1)
	Laparotomy & retroperitoneal biopsy	1	(1)
	Orchidopexy	3	(3)
	Sigmoid resection	1	(1)
	Laparotomy, gastrostomy, duodenectomy	1	(1)
	Inguinal herniotomy	1	(1)
	I & D of abscess	1	(1)
	Hemicolectomy	1	(1)
	Small bowel resection	3	(3)
	Sigmoidoscopy	2	(2)
	Appendicectomy	21	(21)
	I & D pilonidal sinus/abscess	1	(1)
Urgent	Amputation of toe	1	(1)
	Cardioversion	1	(1)
	Sigmoidoscopy	1	(1)
	Exploration of testicles	1	(1)
	Insertion of subclavian line	1	(1)
	OGD	1	(1)
	Incisional hernia repair	1	(1)
	Appendicectomy	11	(11)
	Orchidopexy	1	(1)
	Laparotomy	1	(1)
	Femoral hernia repair	1	(1)
	Repair of bleeding duodenal ulcer	1	(1)
	I & D perianal sepsis	2	(2)
	I & D pilonidal sinus	2	(2)
	I & D abscess	4	(4)
	Small bowel resection	4	(4)
	Sigmoid colectomy & ileostomy	1	
Scheduled	Laparascopic cholecystectomy	1	
	Laparotomy	1	
	Appendicectomy	1	(1)
Elective	Abdoperineal excision of rectum	1	
	I & D abscess	1	
	Excision of skin tags	1	
Blank	Reduction of rectal prolapse	1	(1)
	Removal of foreign body	1	(1)
	Repair of bleeding duodenal ulcer	1	(1)
	Femoral hernia repair	1	(1)
	Laparotomy	1	(1)
	Appendicectomy	2	(2)
	I&D perianal abscess	1	(1)
	I&D abscess	1	(1)

Table 8.12	Gynaecology	

Classification of case	Procedure	Count	
Emergency	EUA & suturing to vaginal vault	1	(1)
	ERPC	7	(7)
	Laparoscopy	2	(2)
	Laparotomy	3	(3)
	Salpingectomy	4	(4)
	EUA – vaginal laceration	1	(1)
	Suction evacuation of uterus	4	(4)
Urgent	Salpingectomy	1	(1)
	Excision ectopic ovarian pregnancy	1	(1)
	ERPC	8	(8)
	Resuturing of wound	1	(1)
	Oophrectomy	1	(1)
	Repair of obstetric tears	1	(1)
	Laparotomy for postoperative bleeding	1	(1)
	ERPC	1	(1)
Elective	Hysteroscopy	1	
Blank	ERPC	1	(1)
	Laparoscopy	1	(1)

Table 8.13	Orthopaedics	

Classification of case	Procedure	Count	
Emergency	Removal of nail from finger	1	(1)
	Intramedullary nail fixation - # tibia	1	(1)
	Internal fixation - # humerus	1	(1)
	Arthroscopy – knee	2	(2)
	Arthroscopy – shoulder	1	(1)
	Reduction and fixation #	1	(1)
	Debride lavage repair compound #	1	(1)
	Reduction and fixation # ankle	2	(2)
	Debridement & suture dog bite	1	(1)
	I&D abscess	1	(1)
	Reduction shoulder dislocation	2	(1)
	Debridement of skin	1	(1)
	Debridement and manipulation # tibia and fibula	2	(2)
	Fasciotomy	1	(1)
	Arthroscopic washout & synovial biopsy	1	(1)
	Reduction of talonavicular joint	1	(1)
	Hemiarthroplasty	2	(2)
	Debridement & manipulation& fixation #knee	1	(1)
	MUA elbow	2	(2)
	Exploration of skin wound	2	
	Reduction & fixation #wrist	1	(1)
Urgent	Open compound fracture tibia & fibula	1	(1)
	Traction – dislocated hip	2	(2)
	Manipulation # finger under anaesthetic	1	(1)
	K wires # bone	1	
	I&D flexor tendosynovitis	1	(1)
	Drainage abscess	2	(2)
	Reduction of fracture – lower end of femur	2	(2)
	Reduction & internal fixation - # ankle	2	(2)
	Dynamic hip screw	1	(1)
	Scaphoid tendon repairs to wrist	1	(1)
	Manipulation # tibia and fibia	1	(1)
	Carpel tunnel decompression	1	(1)
	Debridement open # tibia	1	(1)
	Debridement right hand	1	(1)
	Debridement septic arthritic joint	1	(1)
	Drainage & washout infected knee	1	(1)
	Reduction of # NOF	1	(1)

Table continued overleaf

Table 8.13	Orthopaedics (continued)		
Classification of case	**Procedure**	**Count**	
	Debridement #1st metatarsal	1	(1)
	Fasciotomy	2	(2)
	Manipulation of dislocated shoulder	1	(1)
Scheduled	Spinal fusion	1	
Elective	Arthroscopy	3	(1)
	Lumbar decompression	2	
	Two level discectomy	1	
	Bilateral arthroscopy	1	
	Total hip replacement	6	
	Total knee replacement	5	
	Removal of metalwork	1	
	Carpel tunnel release	1	
Blank	Removal of needle	1	(1)
	Excision cyst	1	(1)
	Exploration of skin wound	1	(1)

Table 8.14	Vascular		
Classification of case	**Procedure**	**Count**	
Emergency	Repair aneurysm	1	(1)
	Closure of femoral artery	1	(1)
	Femoral embolectomy	4	(3)
	Evacuation of retroperitoneal haematoma	1	(1)
	Debridement of diabetic foot	1	(1)
	Aorta unifemoral graft	1	(1)
	Laparotomy	1	(1)
	Gastroscopy	1	(1)
	Calf muscle repair – trauma	1	(1)
Urgent	I&D abscess	1	(1)
	Appendicectomy	1	(1)
	Femoral embolectomy	1	(1)
	Kidney transplant	1	(1)

9 INDEX CASES

INTRODUCTION

Index cases were chosen with the help of the advisors. The index cases included in the report have been chosen to highlight how emergency work is managed in different specialties. Columns and rows that contain no data have been excluded; for example, if an index procedure was never performed at night, the night column has not been included.

Not all returns to NCEPOD were filled in fully. Where this is the case, it has been necessary to exclude these operations from the analysis. Consequently when comparing tables of index operations it will be seen that the totals sometimes differ. Minor differences can also be seen between tables in this chapter and those in the preceding chapter. In some cases this is due to the procedure being able to be performed by more than one specialty.

There is an apparent anomaly of emergency operations being scheduled or performed electively. Some instances may be due to poor reporting but others may be explained by emergencies arising in patients who have been admitted to hospital for other scheduled or elective reasons. An example would be the development of gastrointestinal haemorrhage arising postoperatively in a patient admitted for elective hip joint replacement.

Cardiothoracic surgery

Mitral valve disease

Table 9.1	Count of grade of senior surgeon by time of operation performed during weekdays and weekends					
Grade of surgeon	**Weekday**			**Weekend**		
	Day (%) n=44	Evening (%) n=1	Night (%) n=4	Day (%) n=3	Total (%) n=52	
Consultant	40 (91)	1 (100)	4 (100)	2 (67)	47 (90)	
SAS	1 (2)	0 (0)	0 (0)	0 (0)	1 (2)	
SpR 3 and above	0 (0)	0 (0)	0 (0)	1 (33)	1 (2)	
Blank	3 (7)	0 (0)	0 (0)	0 (0)	3 (6)	

Table 9.2	Count of grade of senior anaesthetist by time of operation performed during weekdays and weekends					
Grade of anaesthetist	**Weekday**			**Weekend**		
	Day (%) n=44	Evening (%) n=1	Night (%) n=4	Day (%) n=3	Total (%) n=52	
Consultant	36 (82)	1 (100)	4 (100)	3 (100)	44 (85)	
SAS	2 (5)	0 (0)	0 (0)	0 (0)	2 (4)	
Other	2 (5)	0 (0)	0 (0)	0 (0)	2 (4)	
Blank	4 (9)	0 (0)	0 (0)	0 (0)	4 (8)	

Table 9.3	Count of classification of theatre case by time during weekdays and weekends					
Classification	**Weekday**			**Weekend**		
	Day (%) n=44	Evening (%) n=1	Night (%) n=4	Day (%) n=3	Total (%) n=52	
Emergency	1 (2)	0 (0)	0 (0)	1 (33)	2 (4)	
Urgent	1 (2)	0 (0)	0 (0)	2 (67)	3 (6)	
Scheduled	16 (36)	0 (0)	0 (0)	0 (0)	16 (31)	
Elective	25 (57)	1 (100)	3 (75)	0 (0)	29 (56)	
Blank	1 (2)	0 (0)	1 (25)	0 (0)	2 (4)	

In this specialty most work is elective or scheduled. Night surgery is now uncommon. Nevertheless, there will always be a need for cardiothoracic surgeons of sufficient seniority and expertise to be available to deal with postoperative complications and trauma to the thoracic viscera. The returns for this specialty demonstrate that consultant surgeons and anaesthetists are present at the majority of operations.

General surgery

Gastrointestinal haemorrhage

Table 9.4	Count of grade of senior surgeon by time of operation performed during weekdays and weekends						
	Weekday			**Weekend**			
Grade of surgeon	**Day (%)** n=29	**Evening (%)** n=16	**Night (%)** n=5	**Day (%)** n=10	**Evening %** n=6	**Night (%)** n=1	**Total (%)** n=67
Consultant	21 (72)	10 (63)	4 (80)	4 (40)	1 (17)	1 (100)	41 (61)
SAS	2 (7)	2 (13)	0 (0)	0 (0)	1 (17)	0 (0)	5 (7)
SpR 1/2	0 (0)	1 (6)	0 (0)	1 (10)	0 (0)	0 (0)	2 (3)
SpR 3 and above	4 (14)	2 (13)	1 (20)	2 (20)	3 (50)	0 (0)	12 (18)
Other	2 (7)	0 (0)	0 (0)	1 (10)	1 (17)	0 (0)	4 (6)
Blank	0 (0)	1 (6)	0 (0)	2 (20)	0 (0)	0 (0)	3 (4)

Table 9.5	Count of grade of senior anaesthetist by time of operation performed during weekdays and weekends						
	Weekday			**Weekend**			
Grade of anaesthetist	**Day (%)** n=29	**Evening (%)** n=16	**Night (%)** n=5	**Day (%)** n=10	**Evening (%)** n=6	**Night (%)** n=1	**Total (%)** n=67
Consultant	20 (69)	11 (69)	2 (40)	4 (40)	0 (0)	0 (0)	37 (55)
SAS	2 (7)	0 (0)	0 (0)	0 (0)	1 (17)	0 (0)	3 (4)
SpR 3 and above	2 (7)	1 (6)	1 (20)	2 (20)	1 (17)	1 (100)	8 (12)
SpR 1/2	0 (0)	0 (0)	0 (0)	1 (10)	0 (0)	0 (0)	1 (1)
SHO	1 (3)	3 (19)	0 (0)	2 (20)	2 (33)	0 (0)	8 (12)
Other	0 (0)	0 (0)	0 (0)	0 (0)	1 (17)	0 (0)	1 (1)
No anaesthetist present	2 (7)	0 (0)	0 (0)	0 (0)	0 (0)	0 (0)	2 (3)
Blank	2 (7)	1 (6)	2 (40)	1 (10)	1 (17)	0 (0)	7 (10)

Table 9.6	Count of classification of theatre case by time during weekdays and weekends						
	Weekday			**Weekend**			
Classification	**Day (%)** n=29	**Evening (%)** n=16	**Night (%)** n=5	**Day (%)** n=10	**Evening (%)** n=6	**Night (%)** n=1	**Total (%)** n=67
Emergency	9 (31)	10 (63)	3 (60)	6 (60)	3 (50)	1 (100)	32 (48)
Urgent	3 (10)	6 (38)	0 (0)	4 (40)	2 (33)	0 (0)	15 (22)
Scheduled	6 (21)	0 (0)	0 (0)	0 (0)	0 (0)	0 (0)	6 (9)
Elective	11 (38)	0 (0)	0 (0)	0 (0)	0 (0)	0 (0)	11 (16)
Blank	0 (0)	0 (0)	2 (40)	0 (0)	1 (17)	0 (0)	3 (4)

A consultant surgeon was present for the majority of these operations, especially during the week, but at the weekend patients were more likely to be operated on by unsupervised junior staff. The trend can also be seen in the grade of anaesthetist present.

Discussion about the management of GI bleeding at the advisors' meetings highlighted the concerns, shared in many specialties, that centralisation of cancer services was leaving increasingly deskilled surgeons in less specialised units to deal with sick and complex cases who may be unfit for transfer.

Continued overleaf

Consultant surgeon:

"The problem with GI bleeding now, from the coal face, is that we are, as surgeons, just getting the residuum of patients that are either not dealt with by the radiologists or the GI physicians with adrenalin injections. So we are getting a very, very high risk group, and they are real crook (sic) patients, and a lot of them die.

*Secondly, if you look at regions that have had a very aggressive policy about centralisation of upper GI cancer services you are starting to see deaths during transfer of unstable patients. There have certainly been two in the ******** region recently, and I think we have to be a little bit careful regarding recommendations about transferring unstable haemorrhaging patients from one place to another."*

Gynaecology

Ectopic pregnancy

Table 9.7	Count of grade of senior surgeon by time of operation performed during weekdays and weekends						
	Weekday			Weekend			
Grade of surgeon	Day (%) n=57	Evening (%) n=44	Night (%) n=8	Day (%) n=13	Evening (%) n=4	Night (%) n=2	Total (%) n=128
Consultant	35 (61)	19 (43)	4 (50)	8 (62)	2 (50)	1 (50)	69 (54)
SAS	6 (11)	2 (5)	2 (25)	1 (8)	1 (25)	1 (50)	13 (10)
SpR 3 and above	2 (4)	6 (14)	0 (0)	2 (15)	1 (25)	0 (0)	11 (9)
SpR 1/2	4 (7)	3 (7)	0 (0)	1 (8)	0 (0)	0 (0)	8 (6)
SHO	0 (0)	2 (5)	1 (13)	0 (0)	0 (0)	0 (0)	3 (2)
Other	4 (7)	9 (20)	1 (13)	1 (8)	0 (0)	0 (0)	15 (12)
Blank	6 (11)	3 (7)	0 (0)	0 (0)	0 (0)	0 (0)	9 (7)

Table 9.8	Count of grade of senior anaesthetist by time of operation performed during weekdays and weekends						
	Weekday			Weekend			
Grade of anaesthetist	Day (%) n=57	Evening (%) n=44	Night (%) n=8	Day (%) n=13	Evening (%) n=4	Night (%) n=2	Total (%) n=128
Consultant	24 (42)	8 (18)	0 (0)	3 (23)	0 (0)	0 (0)	35 (27)
SAS	9 (16)	6 (14)	0 (0)	1 (8)	2 (50)	0 (0)	18 (14)
SpR 3 and above	6 (11)	1 (2)	0 (0)	3 (23)	0 (0)	0 (0)	10 (8)
SpR 1/2	3 (5)	4 (9)	1 (13)	0 (0)	0 (0)	0 (0)	8 (6)
SHO	11 (19)	21 (48)	4 (50)	6 (46)	0 (0)	2 (100)	44 (34)
Other	3 (5)	3 (7)	3 (38)	0 (0)	2 (50)	0 (0)	11 (9)
Blank	1 (2)	1 (2)	0 (0)	0 (0)	0 (0)	0 (0)	2 (2)

Table 9.9	Count of classification of theatre case by time during weekdays and weekends						
	Weekday			Weekend			
Classification	Day (%) n=57	Evening (%) n=44	Night (%) n=8	Day (%) n=13	Evening (%) n=4	Night (%) n=2	Total (%) n=128
Emergency	26 (46)	21 (48)	6 (75)	9 (69)	1 (25)	1 (50)	64 (50)
Urgent	20 (35)	17 (39)	2 (25)	4 (31)	0 (0)	1 (50)	44 (34)
Scheduled	5 (9)	1 (2)	0 (0)	0 (0)	1 (25)	0 (0)	7 (5)
Elective	3 (5)	2 (5)	0 (0)	0 (0)	0 (0)	0 (0)	5 (4)
Blank	3 (5)	3 (7)	0 (0)	0 (0)	2 (50)	0 (0)	8 (6)

During the day and evening most women with an ectopic pregnancy will have an operation performed or supervised by a consultant. During the night it is more likely that the operation will be performed by a more junior grade of surgeon. At all times it is likely that the anaesthetist will be a junior.

Surgery for an ectopic pregnancy is only required at night if there is evidence that the patient is bleeding. If patients operated on at night are genuinely more acute than those operated on during the day it might be expected that the surgical and anaesthetist staff would be of senior grades.

Incomplete miscarriage

Table 9.10	Count of grade of senior surgeon by time of operation performed during weekdays and weekends						
Grade of surgeon	**Weekday**			**Weekend**			
	Day (%) n=37	**Evening (%)** n=18	**Night (%)** n=1	**Day (%)** n=4	**Evening (%)** n=4	**Night (%)** n=2	**Total (%)** n=66
Consultant	11 (30)	1 (6)	0 (0)	0 (0)	2 (50)	0 (0)	**14 (21)**
SAS	3 (8)	1 (6)	0 (0)	0 (0)	0 (0)	1 (50)	**5 (8)**
SpR 3 and above	6 (16)	5 (28)	1 (100)	1 (25)	0 (0)	1 (50)	**14 (21)**
SpR 1/2	10 (27)	2 (11)	0 (0)	1 (25)	1 (25)	0 (0)	**14 (21)**
SHO	3 (8)	2 (11)	0 (0)	2 (50)	1 (25)	0 (0)	**8 (12)**
Other	4 (11)	6 (33)	0 (0)	0 (0)	0 (0)	0 (0)	**10 (15)**
Blank	0 (0)	1 (6)	0 (0)	0 (0)	0 (0)	0 (0)	**1 (2)**

Table 9.11	Count of grade of senior anaesthetist by time of operation performed during weekdays and weekends						
Grade of anaesthetist	**Weekday**			**Weekend**			
	Day (%) n=37	**Evening (%)** n=18	**Night (%)** n=1	**Day (%)** n=4	**Evening (%)** n=4	**Night (%)** n=2	**Total (%)** n=66
Consultant	13 (35)	1 (6)	0 (0)	0 (0)	2 (50)	0 (0)	**16 (24)**
SAS	7 (19)	0 (0)	0 (0)	0 (0)	0 (0)	1 (50)	**8 (12)**
SpR 3 and above	0 (0)	1 (6)	0 (0)	1 (25)	1 (25)	0 (0)	**3 (5)**
SpR 1/2	0 (0)	2 (11)	0 (0)	1 (25)	0 (0)	0 (0)	**3 (5)**
SHO	11 (30)	13 (72)	1 (100)	1 (25)	1 (25)	1 (50)	**28 (42)**
Other	5 (14)	0 (0)	0 (0)	1 (25)	0 (0)	0 (0)	**6 (9)**
Blank	1 (3)	1 (6)	0 (0)	0 (0)	0 (0)	0 (0)	**2 (3)**

Table 9.12	Count of classification of theatre case by time during weekdays and weekends						
Classification	**Weekday**			**Weekend**			
	Day (%) n=37	**Evening (%)** n=18	**Night (%)** n=1	**Day (%)** n=4	**Evening (%)** n=4	**Night (%)** n=2	**Total (%)** n=66
Emergency	13 (35)	9 (50)	1 (100)	2 (50)	1 (25)	2 (100)	**28 (42)**
Urgent	16 (43)	7 (39)	0 (0)	1 (25)	3 (75)	0 (0)	**27 (41)**
Scheduled	4 (11)	0 (0)	0 (0)	0 (0)	0 (0)	0 (0)	**4 (6)**
Elective	3 (8)	0 (0)	0 (0)	0 (0)	0 (0)	0 (0)	**3 (5)**
Blank	1 (3)	2 (11)	0 (0)	1 (25)	0 (0)	0 (0)	**4 (6)**

Compared to ectopic pregnancy, consultant surgeons are less likely to be present when patients undergo surgery for incomplete miscarriage. Most of these patients are however operated on during the day or evening when senior help is most likely to be available.

Maxillofacial surgery

Facial lacerations

Table 9.13	Count of grade of senior surgeon by time of operation performed during weekdays and weekends				
	Weekday		Weekend		
Grade of surgeon	Day (%) n=16	Evening (%) n=8	Day (%) n= 9	Evening (%) n=4	Total (%) n=37
Consultant	3 (19)	1 (13)	2 (22)	2 (50)	8 (22)
SAS	3 (19)	0 (0)	2 (22)	2 (50)	7 (19)
SpR 3 and above	0 (0)	1 (13)	0 (0)	0 (0)	1 (3)
SpR 1/2	2 (13)	2 (25)	2 (22)	0 (0)	6 (16)
SHO	6 (38)	4 (50)	3 (33)	0 (0)	13 (35)
Other	2 (13)	0 (0)	0 (0)	0 (0)	2 (5)
Blank	0 (0)	0 (0)	0 (0)	0 (0)	0 (0)

Table 9.14	Count of grade of senior anaesthetist by time of operation performed during weekdays and weekends				
	Weekday		Weekend		
Grade of anaesthetist	Day (%) n=16	Evening (%) n=8	Day (%) n=9	Evening (%) n=4	Total (%) n=37
Consultant	9 (56)	2 (25)	3 (33)	2 (50)	16 (43)
SAS	1 (6)	1 (13)	0 (0)	0 (0)	2 (5)
SpR 3 and above	1 (6)	1 (13)	3 (33)	2 (50)	7 (19)
SpR1/2	2 (13)	0 (0)	0 (0)	0 (0)	2 (5)
SHO	1 (6)	2 (25)	3 (33)	0 (0)	6 (16)
Other	1 (6)	1 (13)	0 (0)	0 (0)	2 (5)
Blank	1 (6)	1 (13)	0 (0)	0 (0)	2 (5)

Table 9.15	Count of classification of theatre case by time during weekdays and weekends				
	Weekday		Weekend		
Classification	Day (%) n=16	Evening (%) n=8	Day (%) n=9	Evening (%) n=4	Total (%) n=37
Emergency	4 (25)	8 (100)	6 (67)	3 (75)	21 (57)
Urgent	7 (44)	0 (0)	1 (11)	1 (25)	9 (24)
Scheduled	3 (19)	0 (0)	1 (11)	0 (0)	4 (11)
Elective	1 (6)	0 (0)	0 (0)	0 (0)	1 (3)
Blank	1 (6)	0 (0)	1 (11)	0 (0)	2 (5)

Facial lacerations present as emergencies and unless there is life threatening bleeding, do not require immediate surgery. Our advisors suggest that to reduce the risk of infection they should be operated on within 24 hours. It would appear that this condition is being treated appropriately.

Neurosurgery

Spinal compression

Table 9.16	Count of grade of senior surgeon by time of operation performed during weekdays and weekends					
Grade of surgeon	Weekday			Weekend		Total (%) n=51
	Day (%) n=38	Evening (%) n=3	Night (%) n=2	Day (%) n=7	Evening (%) n=1	
Consultant	35 (92)	2 (67)	2 (100)	7 (100)	0 (0)	46 (90)
SpR 3 and above	1 (3)	0 (0)	0 (0)	0 (0)	0 (0)	1 (2)
SpR 1/2	0 (0)	1 (33)	0 (0)	0 (0)	1 (100)	2 (4)
Blank	2 (5)	0 (0)	0 (0)	0 (0)	0 (0)	2 (4)

Table 9.17	Count of grade of senior anaesthetist by time of operation performed during weekdays and weekends					
Grade of anaesthetist	Weekday			Weekend		Total (%) n=51
	Day (%) n=38	Evening (%) n=3	Night (%) n=2	Day (%) n=7	Evening (%) n=1	
Consultant	30 (79)	2 (67)	2 (100)	5 (71)	0 (0)	39 (76)
SAS	4 (11)	0 (0)	0 (0)	2 (29)	0 (0)	6 (12)
SpR 3 and above	2 (5)	1 (33)	0 (0)	0 (0)	0 (0)	3 (6)
SpR 1/2	1 (3)	0 (0)	0 (0)	0 (0)	1 (100)	2 (4)
SHO	1 (3)	0 (0)	0 (0)	0 (0)	0 (0)	1 (2)
Blank	0 (0)	0 (0)	0 (0)	0 (0)	0 (0)	0 (0)

Table 9.18	Count of classification of theatre case by time during weekdays and weekends					
Classification	Weekday			Weekend		Total (%) n=51
	Day (%) n=38	Evening (%) n=3	Night (%) n=2	Day (%) n=7	Evening (%) n=1	
Emergency	0 (0)	2 (67)	0 (0)	1 (14)	0 (0)	3 (6)
Urgent	1 (3)	0 (0)	0 (0)	0 (0)	1 (100)	2 (4)
Scheduled	6 (16)	0 (0)	0 (0)	3 (43)	0 (0)	9 (18)
Elective	29 (76)	1 (33)	2 (100)	3 (43)	0 (0)	35 (69)
Blank	2 (5)	0 (0)	0 (0)	0 (0)	0 (0)	2 (4)

Almost all patients with spinal compression were operated on by consultant surgeons and anaesthetised by consultant or SAS anaesthetists. It is seldom necessary to operate at night. The two cases shown in the table as being performed at night are probably early start elective cases.

Advisors were concerned about the availability of support services.

Consultant surgeon:

"..............management of acute spinal cord compression, particularly in those centres that do not offer a 24 hour MRI service, and that is quite a big issue because I think it is an issue of patient compromise. It has been recognised that patients with central disc prolapses perhaps do not do so well if they do not get decompressed early. Certainly in our unit, which has two spinal surgeons and is regarded as a sort of regional centre, we do not have 24 hour MRI availability, and that is due to apparently staffing shortages and the costs of actually providing the service. I think CEPOD (sic) could make a comment on that because I think that does prejudice patient care, and I would be interested to know what people think."

Consultant surgeon:

"All right, well as far as morbidity is concerned it is entirely true that if someone has significant spinal cord compression with involvement of bladder function they need surgical decompression as soon as it can be arranged, but you have to investigate them first, and that is why most people would agree that MRI scans should be carried out at night. If you do not have the facility for an MRI scan, and you do not have access to it, you can do a myelogram. I think almost every neurosurgical unit that I am aware of does have facilities for myelography and I think that the staffing implications are a little bit different from MRI, though MRI is quicker, it is a more sensible, less invasive procedure and if one were to make recommendations about this I think 24 hour availability of MRI scan is absolutely essential. Do you disagree?"

Consultant radiologist:

"Through most departments in the country, emergency MRI is not available, but I agree with what you said that it should be. That would be a really good way to go forward. What would happen then is that there would be more reasons to do an emergency MRI scan developing in all the other specialties, but most units will run an emergency MRI centre if they are any good."

This issue has been highlighted in the Facilities chapter. Not only should patients have access to timely surgery but they should also have access to appropriate imaging and other investigations.

Paediatric surgery

Torsion of testis

Table 9.19	Count of grade of senior surgeon by time of operation performed during weekdays and weekends					
	Weekday			**Weekend**		
Grade of Surgeon	Day (%) n=4	Evening (%) n=7	Night (%) n=3	Day (%) n=1	Night (%) n=2	Total (%) n=17
Consultant	0 (0)	1 (14)	0 (0)	0 (0)	0 (0)	**1 (6)**
SAS	2 (50)	2 (29)	0 (0)	0 (0)	1 (50)	**5 (29)**
SpR 3 and above	0 (0)	0 (0)	3 (100)	0 (0)	0 (0)	**3 (18)**
SpR 1/2	0 (0)	3 (43)	0 (0)	0 (0)	0 (0)	**3 (18)**
SHO	0 (0)	0 (0)	0 (0)	1 (100)	1 (50)	**2 (12)**
Other	1 (25)	0 (0)	0 (0)	0 (0)	0 (0)	**1 (6)**
Blank	1 (25)	1 (14)	0 (0)	0 (0)	0 (0)	**2 (12)**

Table 9.20	Count of grade of senior anaesthetist by time of operation performed during weekdays and weekends					
	Weekday			**Weekend**		
Grade of anaesthetist	Day (%) n=4	Evening (%) n=7	Night (%) n=3	Day (%) n=1	Night (%) n=2	Total (%) n=17
Consultant	1 (25)	0 (0)	0 (0)	0 (0)	1 (50)	**2 (12)**
SAS	2 (50)	0 (0)	0 (0)	1 (100)	0 (0)	**3 (18)**
SpR 3 and above	0 (0)	1 (14)	2 (67)	0 (0)	0 (0)	**3 (18)**
SpR 1/2	0 (0)	1 (14)	0 (0)	0 (0)	0 (0)	**1 (6)**
SHO	1 (25)	5 (71)	1 (33)	0 (0)	1 (50)	**8 (47)**
Blank	0 (0)	0 (0)	0 (0)	0 (0)	0 (0)	**0 (0)**

Table 9.21	Count of classification of theatre case by time during weekdays and weekends					
	Weekday			**Weekend**		
Classification	Day (%) n=4	Evening (%) n=7	Night (%) n=3	Day (%) n=1	Night (%) n=2	Total (%) n=17
Emergency	4 (100)	5 (71)	2 (67)	1 (100)	1 (50)	**13 (76)**
Urgent	0 (0)	2 (29)	1 (33)	0 (0)	1 (50)	**4 (24)**
Blank	0 (0)	0 (0)	0 (0)	0 (0)	0 (0)	**0 (0)**

While torsion of the testis is not life threatening it is generally accepted that urgent surgery is required if a potentially viable testis is to be saved. This highlights one of the deficiencies of the NCEPOD classification of cases which we have earlier recommended should be reviewed. This is not a life threatening condition. However, it would be negligent to wait up to 24 hours for an operation on torsion of the testis.

Consultant surgeon:

"Then there is torsion of testis which, of course, does not lead to the death of a child but to the loss of a testis, and we would crash lists for that, routinely, if we were operating. We would stop the next available list and do a torsion when we do not have a CEPOD (sic) list."

Plastic surgery

Tendon damage

Table 9.22	Count of grade of senior surgeon by time of operation performed during weekdays and weekends				
Grade of surgeon	**Weekday**		**Weekend**		**Total (%)** n=137
	Day (%) n=79	**Evening (%)** n=23	**Day (%)** n=29	**Evening (%)** n=6	
Consultant	26 (33)	2 (9)	2 (7)	0 (0)	**30 (22)**
SAS	6 (8)	0 (0)	4 (14)	0 (0)	**10 (7)**
SpR 3 and above	17 (22)	9 (39)	8 (28)	2 (33)	**36 (26)**
SpR 1/2	15 (19)	7 (30)	6 (21)	2 (33)	**30 (22)**
SHO	4 (5)	1 (4)	1 (3)	0 (0)	**6 (4)**
Other	11 (14)	4 (17)	8 (28)	2 (33)	**25 (18)**
Blank	0 (0)	0 (0)	0 (0)	0 (0)	**0 (0)**

Table 9.23	Count of grade of senior anaesthetist by time of operation performed during weekdays and weekends				
Grade of anaesthetist	**Weekday**		**Weekend**		**Total (%)** n=137
	Day (%) n=79	**Evening (%)** n=23	**Day (%)** n=29	**Evening (%)** n=6	
Consultant	26 (33)	5 (22)	2 (7)	1 (17)	**34 (25)**
SAS	4 (5)	0 (0)	3 (10)	0 (0)	**7 (5)**
SpR 3 and above	4 (5)	3 (13)	6 (21)	1 (17)	**14 (10)**
SpR 1/2	8 (10)	2 (9)	1 (3)	0 (0)	**11 (8)**
SHO	4 (5)	5 (22)	7 (24)	2 (33)	**18 (13)**
Other	4 (5)	4 (17)	3 (10)	1 (17)	**12 (9)**
No anaesthetist present	16 (20)	1 (4)	5 (17)	0 (0)	**22 (16)**
Blank	13 (16)	3 (13)	2 (7)	1 (17)	**19 (14)**

Table 9.24	Count of classification of theatre case by time during weekdays and weekends				
Classification	**Weekday**		**Weekend**		**Total (%)** n=137
	Day n=79	**Evening (%)** n=23	**Day (%)** n=29	**Evening (%)** n=6	
Emergency	27 (34)	9 (39)	16 (55)	1 (17)	**53 (39)**
Urgent	19 (24)	12 (52)	10 (34)	2 (33)	**43 (31)**
Scheduled	7 (9)	0 (0)	1 (3)	1 (17)	**9 (7)**
Elective	20 (25)	0 (0)	1 (3)	1 (17)	**22 (16)**
Blank	6 (8)	2 (9)	1 (3)	1 (17)	**10 (7)**

Primary tendon repair is an urgent procedure performed primarily by plastic and orthopaedic surgeons. There is no need for the procedure to be performed at night.

Continued overleaf

Consultant surgeon:

"Interestingly, primary tendon repair is not a true emergency in the way it is classified in the questionnaire, but quite a lot of them have been classified as emergencies. Only a few were done in the evening, which is probably about right, so I think they are getting done at the right time, they are not being done in the middle of the night, so that is correct. None at all, I think, from this were done at night."

NCEPOD clinical co-ordinator:

"Would you say extensor tendons were as urgent as flexors?"

Consultant surgeon:

"I would say it is the same, really, I would effectively count them as the same."

Trauma/Orthopaedic surgery

Fractured neck of femur

Table 9.25	Count of grade of senior surgeon by time of operation performed during weekdays and weekends						
	Weekday			Weekend			
Grade of surgeon	Day (%) n=485	Evening (%) n=32	Night (%) n=3	Day (%) n=187	Evening (%) n=16	Night (%) n=2	Total (%) n=725
Consultant	181 (37)	5 (16)	2 (67)	38 (20)	4 (25)	0 (0)	230 (32)
SAS	113 (23)	5 (16)	0 (0)	43 (23)	3 (19)	0 (0)	164 (23)
SpR 3 and above	70 (14)	8 (25)	0 (0)	43 (23)	6 (38)	0 (0)	127 (18)
SpR 1/2	47 (10)	5 (16)	1 (33)	36 (19)	2 (13)	2 (100)	93 (13)
SHO	9 (2)	3 (9)	0 (0)	3 (2)	0 (0)	0 (0)	15 (2)
Other	37 (8)	5 (16)	0 (0)	15 (8)	0 (0)	0 (0)	57 (8)
Blank	28 (6)	1 (3)	0 (0)	9 (5)	1 (6)	0 (0)	39 (5)

Table 9.26	Count of grade of senior anaesthetist by time of operation performed during weekdays and weekends						
	Weekday			Weekend			
Grade of anaesthetist	Day (%) n=485	Evening (%) n=32	Night (%) n=3	Day (%) n=187	Evening (%) n=16	Night (%) n=2	Total (%) n=725
Consultant	266 (55)	8 (25)	2 (67)	45 (24)	0 (0)	0 (0)	321 (44)
SAS	92 (19)	9 (28)	0 (0)	37 (20)	1 (6)	0 (0)	139 (19)
SpR 3 and above	23 (5)	1 (3)	0 (0)	21 (11)	3 (19)	0 (0)	48 (7)
SpR 1/2	15 (3)	1 (3)	0 (0)	7 (4)	1 (6)	0 (0)	24 (3)
SHO	37 (8)	9 (28)	1 (33)	57 (30)	10 (63)	2 (100)	116 (16)
Other	35 (7)	3 (9)	0 (0)	15 (8)	1 (6)	0 (0)	54 (7)
No anaesthetist present	1 (0)	0 (0)	0 (0)	0 (0)	0 (0)	0 (0)	1 (0)
Blank	16 (3)	1 (3)	0 (0)	5 (3)	0 (0)	0 (0)	22 (3)

Table 9.27	Count of classification of theatre case by time during weekdays and weekends						
	Weekday			Weekend			
Classification	Day (%) n=485	Evening (%) n=32	Night (%) n=3	Day (%) n=187	Evening (%) n=16	Night (%) n=2	Total (%) n=725
Emergency	97 (20)	9 (28)	1 (33)	60 (32)	3 (19)	1 (50)	171 (24)
Urgent	214 (44)	14 (44)	2 (67)	97 (52)	11 (69)	1 (50)	339 (47)
Scheduled	84 (17)	3 (9)	0 (0)	19 (10)	1 (6)	0 (0)	107 (15)
Elective	38 (8)	1 (3)	0 (0)	0 (0)	0 (0)	0 (0)	39 (5)
Blank	52 (11)	5 (16)	0 (0)	11 (6)	1 (6)	0 (0)	69 (10)

Again, we see a pattern of consultant surgeons and anaesthetists being involved more often when patients are operated on during the week especially between 08:00 and 18:00. Is there any evidence that patients operated on by more junior staff are any less complex? Or do the working patterns reflect the fact that there are only enough consultants to staff lists during the day? There are guidelines suggesting that surgery for fractured neck of femur should be carried out within 24 hours and during standard daytime working hours (including weekends) if the patient's condition permits. [22,23]

Continued overleaf

Forearm fracture

Table 9.28	Count of grade of senior surgeon by time of operation performed during weekdays and weekends				
Grade of surgeon	**Weekday**		**Weekend**		**Total (%)** n=293
	Day (%) n=149	**Evening (%)** n=58	**Day (%)** n=57	**Evening (%)** n=29	
Consultant	56 (38)	7 (12)	17 (30)	2 (7)	82 (28)
SAS	39 (26)	13 (22)	14 (25)	4 (14)	70 (24)
SpR 3 and above	17 (11)	11 (19)	10 (18)	10 (34)	48 (16)
SpR 1/2	18 (12)	9 (16)	9 (16)	8 (28)	44 (15)
SHO	6 (4)	2 (3)	1 (2)	1 (3)	10 (3)
Other	10 (7)	13 (22)	5 (9)	3 (10)	31 (11)
Blank	3 (2)	3 (5)	1 (2)	1 (3)	8 (3)

Table 9.29	Count of grade of senior anaesthetist by time of operation performed during weekdays and weekends				
Grade of anaesthetist	**Weekday**		**Weekend**		**Total (%)** n=293
	Day (%) n=149	**Evening (%)** n=58	**Day (%)** n=57	**Evening (%)** n=29	
Consultant	72 (48)	9 (16)	11 (19)	1 (3)	93 (32)
SAS	25 (17)	9 (16)	12 (21)	1 (3)	47 (16)
SpR 3 and above	9 (6)	7 (12)	5 (9)	3 (10)	24 (8)
SpR 1/2	9 (6)	1 (2)	7 (12)	7 (24)	24 (8)
SHO	18 (12)	22 (38)	18 (32)	14 (48)	72 (25)
Other	12 (8)	8 (14)	1 (2)	3 (10)	24 (8)
Blank	4 (3)	2 (3)	3 (5)	0 (0)	9 (3)

Table 9.30	Count of classification of theatre case by time during weekdays and weekends				
Classification	**Weekday**		**Weekend**		**Total (%)** n=293
	Day (%) n=149	**Evening (%)** n=58	**Day (%)** n=57	**Evening (%)** n=29	
Emergency	28 (19)	26 (45)	26 (46)	14 (48)	94 (32)
Urgent	74 (50)	25 (43)	26 (46)	13 (45)	138 (47)
Scheduled	29 (19)	2 (3)	4 (7)	1 (3)	36 (12)
Elective	2 (1)	0 (0)	0 (0)	0 (0)	2 (1)
Blank	16 (11)	5 (9)	1 (2)	1 (3)	23 (8)

This procedure is commonly performed during the day or evening. A consultant performs or supervises the procedure in about a third of cases and there is a similar level of involvement of consultant anaesthetists. Children's fractures are often manipulated out of hours. There is no good evidence that it is necessary for these to be done at night unless there is neurovascular compromise. In fact, in the present study no case was performed at night.

Consultant surgeon:

"The forearm fracture analysis, the manipulation of fracture of the forearm in a child is a procedure that rarely needs to be done at night. It is interesting, when we look down the list, how many of these were done as emergencies or out of hours. There might be an argument that those should not really be done out of hours."

NCEPOD clinical co-ordinator:

"Maybe they need better pain management not a trip to theatre. Would that be correct?"

Consultant surgeon:

"Absolutely. There is quite a lot of literature now which suggests, for example, things like supracondylar fractures of the humerus very, very rarely need to be done as emergencies."

SpR surgeon:

"There are certainly a number of papers that have been produced to that effect. You can certainly wait until the following morning, and it is probably best to do them in the morning with the appropriate staff."

Again this raises the problem of case classification. An open fracture needs to be treated more urgently than a closed fracture.

Vascular surgery

Leaking / ruptured abdominal aortic aneurysm

Table 9.31	Count of grade of senior surgeon by time of operation performed during weekdays and weekends					
	Weekday			Weekend		
Grade of surgeon	Day (%) n=56	Evening (%) n=4	Night (%) n=1	Day (%) n=3	Night (%) n=1	Total (%) n=65
Consultant	54 (96)	4 (100)	1 (100)	3 (100)	1 (100)	63 (97)
Other	1 (2)	0 (0)	0 (0)	0 (0)	0 (0)	1 (2)
Blank	1 (2)	0 (0)	0 (0)	0 (0)	0 (0)	1 (2)

Table 9.32	Count of grade of senior anaesthetist by time of operation performed during weekdays and weekends					
	Weekday			Weekend		
Grade of anaesthetist	Day (%) n=56	Evening (%) n=4	Night (%) n=1	Day (%) n=3	Night (%) n=1	Total (%) n=65
Consultant	51 (91)	4 (100)	0 (0)	2 (67)	1 (100)	58 (89)
SpR 3 and above	1 (2)	0 (0)	1 (100)	1 (33)	0 (0)	3 (5)
SHO	2 (4)	0 (0)	0 (0)	0 (0)	0 (0)	2 (3)
Blank	2 (4)	0 (0)	0 (0)	0 (0)	0 (0)	2 (3)

Table 9.33	Count of classification of theatre case by time during weekdays and weekends					
	Weekday			Weekend		
Classification	Day (%) n=56	Evening (%) n=4	Night (%) n=1	Day (%) n=3	Night (%) n=1	Total (%) n=65
Emergency	11 (20)	4 (100)	1 (100)	3 (100)	1 (100)	20 (31)
Urgent	3 (5)	0 (0)	0 (0)	0 (0)	0 (0)	3 (5)
Scheduled	9 (16)	0 (0)	0 (0)	0 (0)	0 (0)	9 (14)
Elective	26 (46)	0 (0)	0 (0)	0 (0)	0 (0)	26 (40)
Blank	7 (13)	0 (0)	0 (0)	0 (0)	0 (0)	7 (11)

In contrast to many other procedures, patients who present as emergencies with abdominal aortic aneurysms are almost exclusively operated on or under the guidance of a consultant surgeon and anaesthetist. This reflects the life threatening nature of this condition. There can be little argument that surgery should be performed as soon as possible. There were some concerns among the advisors that patients might be disadvantaged if a specialist consultant vascular surgeon was not available especially in the smaller hospitals.

Consultant surgeon:

"I think there is a difference according to whether these are managed in more general units or specialist vascular units, because a lot of the cases managed in specialist vascular units are people who actually have tender aneurysms and they are fit and stable for transfer. Of course, the outcome for those patients is quite different compared to those who are unstable and need emergency procedure, often by a non-vascular surgeon in the middle of the night."

NCEPOD clinical co-ordinator:

"There is almost a triage going on where the worst cases are dealt with in the most inappropriate place."

Consultant surgeon:

"Indeed, by the least experienced surgeons, yes. They may be consultants, but you know, they may be someone like me who does not do any elective vascular surgery at all."

NCEPOD clinical co-ordinator:

"They are not doing elective aneurysms routinely during the week, but they are being expected to deal with the worst of the ruptured aneurysms in an emergency setting."

Consultant surgeon:

"Usually with an entirely predictable outcome!"

Organ failure requiring transplant

| Table 9.34 | Count of grade of senior surgeon by time of operation performed during weekdays and weekends |

Grade of surgeon	Weekday			Weekend			Total (%) n=22
	Day (%) n=12	Evening (%) n=2	Night (%) n=4	Day (%) n=2	Evening (%) n=1	Night (%) n=1	
Consultant	10 (83)	2 (100)	3 (75)	2 (100)	0 (0)	1 (100)	18 (82)
Other	1 (8)	0 (0)	0 (0)	0 (0)	0 (0)	0 (0)	1 (5)
Blank	1 (8)	0 (0)	1 (25)	0 (0)	1 (100)	0 (0)	3 (14)

| Table 9.35 | Count of grade of senior anaesthetist by time of operation performed during weekdays and weekends |

Grade of anaesthetist	Weekday			Weekend			Total (%) n=22
	Day (%) n=12	Evening (%) n=2	Night (%) n=4	Day (%) n=2	Evening (%) n=1	Night (%) n=1	
Consultant	6 (50)	1 (50)	2 (50)	2 (100)	0 (0)	0 (0)	11 (50)
SpR 3 and above	4 (33)	0 (0)	1 (25)	0 (0)	0 (0)	1 (100)	6 (27)
SHO	1 (8)	0 (0)	0 (0)	0 (0)	0 (0)	0 (0)	1 (5)
Other	1 (8)	1 (50)	0 (0)	0 (0)	0 (0)	0 (0)	2 (9)
Blank	0 (0)	0 (0)	1 (25)	0 (0)	1 (100)	0 (0)	2 (9)

| Table 9.36 | Count of classification of theatre case by time during weekdays and weekends |

Classification	Weekday			Weekend			Total (%) n=22
	Day (%) n=12	Evening (%) n=2	Night (%) n=4	Day (%) n=2	Evening (%) n=1	Night (%) n=1	
Emergency	1 (8)	1 (50)	2 (50)	1 (50)	1 (100)	1 (100)	7 (32)
Urgent	2 (17)	1 (50)	1 (25)	0 (0)	0 (0)	0 (0)	4 (18)
Scheduled	2 (17)	0 (0)	0 (0)	0 (0)	0 (0)	0 (0)	2 (9)
Elective	7 (58)	0 (0)	0 (0)	0 (0)	0 (0)	0 (0)	7 (32)
Blank	0 (0)	0 (0)	1 (25)	1 (50)	0 (0)	0 (0)	2 (9)

The timing of retrieval and transplantation of organs must often be managed around access to theatre and staff at two sites. With time constraints on the viability of explanted organs and the possibility that there may be more than one recipient from one donor, it is clear that these operations may need to take place at any time day or night. Procedures involving live related donors can however be scheduled.

Transplantation is funded separately from other surgery and Trusts should ensure that the service is adequately provided for, to reduce the impact that emergency transplant procedures can have on timely surgery for other patients admitted as emergencies.

Acute appendicitis

Because appendicectomy is such a frequently performed emergency operation it is presented in more detail here than the other index procedures.

Table 9.37	Appendicectomy analysis by procedure					
	Age					**Total**
	>=16	**5 – 15**	**0 - 4**	**Blank**		
Conventional	478	200	4	14		**696**
Laparoscopy	49	10	1	0		**60**
Laparotomy	43	1	1	1		**46**
Total	**570**	**211**	**6**	**15**		**802**

Acute appendicitis (All)

Table 9.38	Count of grade of senior surgeon by time of operation performed during weekdays and weekends						
	Weekday			**Weekend**			
Grade of surgeon	**Day (%)** n=322	**Evening (%)** n=254	**Night (%)** n=33	**Day (%)** n=104	**Evening (%)** n=72	**Night (%)** n=17	**Total (%)** n=802
Consultant	117 (36)	36 (14)	3 (9)	21 (20)	5 (7)	2 (12)	**184 (23)**
SAS	35 (11)	50 (20)	4 (12)	14 (13)	14 (19)	2 (12)	**119 (15)**
SpR 3 and above	46 (14)	49 (19)	8 (24)	17 (16)	15 (21)	3 (18)	**138 (17)**
SpR 1/2	51 (16)	38 (15)	6 (18)	20 (19)	11 (15)	6 (35)	**132 (16)**
SHO	18 (6)	28 (11)	1 (3)	14 (13)	10 (14)	2 (12)	**73 (9)**
Other	38 (12)	40 (16)	6 (18)	14 (13)	14 (19)	1 (6)	**113 (14)**
Blank	17 (5)	13 (5)	5 (15)	4 (4)	3 (4)	1 (6)	**43 (5)**

Table 9.39	Count of grade of senior anaesthetist by time of operation performed during weekdays and weekends						
	Weekday			**Weekend**			
Grade of anaesthetist	**Day (%)** n=322	**Evening (%)** n=254	**Night (%)** n=33	**Day (%)** n=104	**Evening (%)** n=72	**Night (%)** n=17	**Total (%)** n=802
Consultant	151 (47)	36 (14)	3 (9)	20 (19)	5 (7)	1 (6)	**216 (27)**
SAS	36 (11)	23 (9)	0 (0)	17 (16)	4 (6)	0 (0)	**80 (10)**
SpR 3 and above	15 (5)	19 (7)	2 (6)	7 (7)	13 (18)	1 (6)	**57 (7)**
SpR1/2	14 (4)	15 (6)	4 (12)	6 (6)	5 (7)	2 (12)	**46 (6)**
SHO	79 (25)	128 (50)	19 (58)	40 (38)	36 (50)	13 (76)	**315 (39)**
Other	19 (6)	19 (7)	4 (12)	8 (8)	4 (6)	0 (0)	**54 (7)**
Blank	8 (2)	14 (6)	1 (3)	6 (6)	5 (7)	0 (0)	**34 (4)**

Continued overleaf

Table 9.40	Count of classification of theatre case by time during weekdays and weekends						
Classification	**Weekday**			**Weekend**			**Total (%)** n=802
	Day (%) n=322	**Evening (%)** n=254	**Night (%)** n=33	**Day (%)** n=104	**Evening (%)** n=72	**Night (%)** n=17	
Emergency	124 (39)	134 (53)	19 (58)	51 (49)	39 (54)	10 (59)	**377 (47)**
Urgent	114 (35)	101 (40)	9 (27)	43 (41)	25 (35)	5 (29)	**297 (37)**
Scheduled	28 (9)	6 (2)	0 (0)	3 (3)	1 (1)	1 (6)	**39 (5)**
Elective	36 (11)	2 (1)	1 (3)	3 (3)	0 (0)	0 (0)	**42 (5)**
Blank	20 (6)	11 (4)	4 (12)	4 (4)	7 (10)	1 (6)	**47 (6)**

We received information on more than 800 patients who underwent appendicectomy. Of note is how often a consultant surgeon was present and how infrequently the procedure is left to an SHO to perform. This represents a change since our previous report. There are probably a number of factors driving this change but it does not appear to be related to an increase in the number of procedures performed laparoscopically which amount to only 10% of all appendicectomies.

SHOs in anaesthetics are however very much involved in the management of these patients. The majority of patients with appendicitis are relatively young and fit and can be safely anaesthetised by a proficient SHO. It would seem that the operation itself is now thought to be beyond the training of most surgical SHOs. This is probably related to restructuring of surgical training. Surgical SHOs are spending less time in theatre than previously.

NCEPOD clinical co-ordinator:

"We have taken on board the difference by what we mean by "registrar" these days because we no longer have senior registrars, so SpRs are what used to be registrars. The trouble is that some registrars are what used to be SHOs, because the registrars that we are appointing now, certainly in log book terms, are often very less experienced than people who were SHOs in a previous time.

I think that is very important because the anaesthetic SHOs at least think they run the hospital at night and usually give as a reason for not doing an appendicectomy is that CEPOD (sic) said you do not do appendicectomies at night. It is not what we said at all, but obviously the impression is that an appendicectomy and appendicitis is a relatively benign condition so there is never any need to do it in the middle of the night - there rarely is, but there is sometimes."

Acute appendicitis (>=16 years of age)

Table 9.41	Count of grade of senior surgeon by time of operation performed during weekdays and weekends

| Grade of surgeon | Weekday | | | Weekend | | | Total (%) n=570 |
	Day (%) n=250	Evening (%) n=165	Night (%) n=22	Day (%) n=69	Evening (%) n=51	Night (%) n=13	
Consultant	92 (37)	23 (14)	2 (9)	15 (22)	4 (8)	1 (8)	137 (24)
SAS	29 (12)	35 (21)	3 (14)	8 (12)	9 (18)	1 (8)	85 (15)
SpR 3 and above	40 (16)	31 (19)	6 (27)	13 (19)	11 (22)	2 (15)	103 (18)
SpR 1/2	36 (14)	23 (14)	3 (14)	14 (20)	10 (20)	5 (38)	91 (16)
SHO	11 (4)	20 (12)	1 (5)	10 (14)	5 (10)	2 (15)	49 (9)
Other	27 (11)	26 (16)	5 (23)	7 (10)	10 (20)	1 (8)	76 (13)
Blank	15 (6)	7 (4)	2 (9)	2 (3)	2 (4)	1 (8)	29 (5)

Table 9.42	Count of grade of senior anaesthetist by time of operation performed during weekdays and weekends

| Grade of Anaesthetist | Weekday | | | Weekend | | | Total (%) n=570 |
	Day (%) n=250	Evening (%) n=165	Night (%) n=22	Day (%) n=69	Evening (%) n=51	Night (%) n=13	
Consultant	117 (47)	23 (14)	1 (5)	12 (17)	5 (10)	0 (0)	158 (28)
SAS	29 (12)	15 (9)	0 (0)	9 (13)	3 (6)	0 (0)	56 (10)
SpR 3 and above	10 (4)	7 (4)	1 (5)	5 (7)	9 (18)	1 (8)	33 (6)
SpR 1/2	8 (3)	10 (6)	2 (9)	4 (6)	3 (6)	2 (15)	29 (5)
SHO	63 (25)	88 (53)	13 (59)	31 (45)	26 (51)	10 (77)	231 (41)
Other	16 (6)	12 (7)	4 (18)	4 (6)	1 (2)	0 (0)	37 (6)
Blank	7 (3)	10 (6)	1 (5)	4 (6)	4 (8)	0 (0)	26 (5)

Table 9.43	Count of classification of theatre case by time during weekdays and weekends

| Classification | Weekday | | | Weekend | | | Total (%) n=570 |
	Day (%) n=250	Evening (%) n=165	Night (%) n=22	Day (%) n=69	Evening (%) n=51	Night (%) n=13	
Emergency	92 (37)	89 (54)	9 (41)	34 (49)	27 (53)	6 (46)	257 (45)
Urgent	88 (35)	63 (38)	8 (36)	26 (38)	19 (37)	5 (38)	209 (37)
Scheduled	23 (9)	6 (4)	0 (0)	2 (3)	1 (2)	1 (8)	33 (6)
Elective	33 (13)	1 (1)	1 (5)	3 (4)	0 (0)	0 (0)	38 (7)
Blank	14 (6)	6 (4)	4 (18)	4 (6)	4 (8)	1 (8)	33 (6)

Continued overleaf

Acute appendicitis (Between 5 and 15 years of age)

Table 9.44	Count of grade of senior surgeon by time of operation performed during weekdays and weekends						
Grade of surgeon	**Weekday**			**Weekend**			
	Day (%) n=66	Evening (%) n=82	Night (%) n=10	Day (%) n=30	Evening (%) n=20	Night (%) n=3	Total (%) n=211
Consultant (paediatric)	9 (14)	1 (1)	0 (0)	1 (3)	0 (0)	0 (0)	11 (5)
Consultant (other)	14 (21)	10 (12)	1 (10)	2 (7)	1 (5)	0 (0)	28 (13)
SAS	6 (9)	14 (17)	1 (10)	6 (20)	5 (25)	1 (33)	33 (16)
SpR 3 and above	6 (9)	18 (22)	2 (20)	4 (13)	3 (15)	1 (33)	34 (16)
SpR 1/2	14 (21)	14 (17)	2 (20)	6 (20)	1 (5)	1 (33)	38 (18)
SHO	6 (9)	8 (10)	0 (0)	4 (13)	5 (25)	0 (0)	23 (11)
Other	9 (14)	13 (16)	1 (10)	6 (20)	4 (20)	0 (0)	33 (16)
Blank	2 (3)	4 (5)	3 (30)	1 (3)	1 (5)	0 (0)	11 (5)

Table 9.45	Count of grade of senior anaesthetist by time of operation performed during weekdays and weekends						
Grade of anaesthetist	**Weekday**			**Weekend**			
	Day (%) n=66	Evening (%) n=82	Night (%) n=10	Day (%) n=30	Evening (%) n=20	Night (%) n=3	Total (%) n=211
Consultant	32 (48)	12 (15)	2 (20)	5 (17)	0 (0)	0 (0)	51 (24)
SAS	7 (11)	7 (9)	0 (0)	7 (23)	1 (5)	0 (0)	22 (10)
SpR 3 and above	5 (8)	11 (13)	1 (10)	2 (7)	4 (20)	0 (0)	23 (11)
SpR 1/2	4 (6)	5 (6)	1 (10)	1 (3)	2 (10)	0 (0)	13 (6)
SHO	15 (23)	36 (44)	6 (60)	9 (30)	9 (45)	3 (100)	78 (37)
Other	3 (5)	7 (9)	0 (0)	4 (13)	3 (15)	0 (0)	17 (8)
Blank	0 (0)	4 (5)	0 (0)	2 (7)	1 (5)	0 (0)	7 (3)

Table 9.46	Count of classification of theatre case by time during weekdays and weekends						
Classification	**Weekday**			**Weekend**			
	Day (%) n=66	Evening (%) n=82	Night (%) n=10	Day (%) n=30	Evening (%) n=20	Night (%) n=3	Total (%) n=211
Emergency	30 (45)	43 (52)	9 (90)	13 (43)	11 (55)	3 (100)	109 (52)
Urgent	26 (39)	33 (40)	1 (10)	17 (57)	6 (30)	0 (0)	83 (39)
Scheduled	4 (6)	0 (0)	0 (0)	0 (0)	0 (0)	0 (0)	4 (2)
Elective	2 (3)	1 (1)	0 (0)	0 (0)	0 (0)	0 (0)	3 (1)
Blank	4 (6)	5 (6)	0 (0)	0 (0)	3 (15)	0 (0)	12 (6)

Acute appendicitis (<5 years of age)

Table 9.47	Count of grade of senior surgeon by time of operation performed during weekdays and weekends				
Grade of surgeon	**Weekday**			**Weekend**	**Total (%)** n=6
	Day (%) n=3	**Evening (%)** n=1	**Night (%)** n=1	**Day (%)** n=1	
Consultant (paediatric)	2 (67)	1 (100)	0 (0)	0 (0)	**3 (50)**
Consultant (other)	0 (0)	0 (0)	0 (0)	1 (100)	**1 (17)**
SpR 1/2	1 (33)	0 (0)	1 (100)	0 (0)	**2 (33)**
Blank	0 (0)	0 (0)	0 (0)	0 (0)	**0 (0)**

Table 9.48	Count of grade of senior anaesthetist by time of operation performed during weekdays and weekends				
Grade of anaesthetist	**Weekday**			**Weekend**	**Total (%)** n=6
	Day (%) n=3	**Evening (%)** n=1	**Night (%)** n=1	**Day (%)** n=1	
Consultant	2 (67)	1 (100)	0 (0)	1 (100)	**4 (67)**
SpR 1/2	1 (33)	0 (0)	1 (100)	0 (0)	**2 (33)**
Blank	0 (0)	0 (0)	0 (0)	0 (0)	**0 (0)**

Table 9.49	Count of classification of theatre case by time during weekdays and weekends				
Classification	**Weekday**			**Weekend**	**Total (%)** n=6
	Day (%) n=3	**Evening (%)** n=1	**Night (%)** n=1	**Day (%)** n=1	
Emergency	1 (33)	1 (100)	1 (100)	1 (100)	**4 (67)**
Elective	1 (33)	0 (0)	0 (0)	0 (0)	**1 (17)**
Blank	1 (33)	0 (0)	0 (0)	0 (0)	**1 (17)**

Children Age 5-15 operated on by paediatric surgeon: 11/211.

Children Age 0-4 operated on by paediatric surgeon: 3/6.

Under the age of 16 years, only a small proportion (5%) of appendicectomies are performed by paediatric surgeons. One should remember that there are many fewer paediatric surgeons than general surgeons and there is a perception among the advisors that there is an increasing trend to refer children to specialist units. This may put a burden on these units that is difficult to cope with. The need to "stem the flow of the general surgery of childhood out of district general hospitals into specialist paediatric surgical units that are having difficulty coping" has been recognised by the SAC in general surgery. [24]

10 DEATHS REPORTED TO NCEPOD

INTRODUCTION

Consistent with previous annual data collection, all deaths occurring in hospitals within 30 days of a surgical procedure, performed by a surgeon or gynaecologist during 2001/02, were requested by NCEPOD. This chapter provides an overview of these cases. Unlike previous NCEPOD studies, the data was not sampled, and was collected separately to the data in the preceding chapters. However, some interesting observations from the data can still be made.

DATA COLLECTION

The data collection period at NCEPOD runs on a financial year basis and the data presented here reports deaths occurring between 1st April 2001 and 31st March 2002.

A nominated local reporter in each hospital reports data on deaths to NCEPOD. Often local reporters report for more than one hospital and their hard work is greatly appreciated. Historically, histopathologists have filled this role as they had the best knowledge and access to data on deaths occurring in their hospital. However, with the increased availability of such data on patient administration systems (PAS) we are now finding that many of the local reporter roles are being transferred to people in clinical governance and information departments. This change benefits NCEPOD as it facilitates our move away from submission of data on hand written forms and towards a preferred method of electronic submission using a spreadsheet. Information departments are much better placed to download and manipulate the data from their hospital PAS.

The method of reporting deaths following surgery using a standard format has been used since NCEPOD started although we cannot take credit for this method as it actually precedes NCEPOD by some 130 years. Florence Nightingale originally described this method in 1859 [25]. Her 'model forms' were designed to ascertain hospital mortality in different hospitals in different regions of the country, although one would assume that the surgical procedures have evolved somewhat since then. As mentioned in previous reports it is now mandatory for all hospitals, including the private sector, to participate in the work of the confidential enquiries [26,27,28]. However, despite updates to medical directors on a quarterly basis, indicating the number of deaths reported from their hospital/s, there are a number of hospitals/Trusts that still fail to send us data during the allocated collection period. Appendix A displays the number of deaths from 2001/02 compared with 2000/01 by hospital/Trust.

Data related to deaths are requested by NCEPOD from all NHS hospitals in England, Wales and Northern Ireland. Data are also reported from Guernsey, Jersey, the Isle of Man, Defence Secondary Care Agency and the majority of the independent sector. Data was not collected from Scotland where the Scottish Audit of Surgical Mortality (SASM) performs a similar function.

ANALYSIS OF THE DATA

In the original 'Who Operates When?' report of 1995/96 (WOW I), no analysis was performed on the reported deaths. A summary of the number of deaths by region was described, although due to ever changing regional boundaries a direct comparison cannot be made with this year's data. However, the total number of 19,841 deaths reported in 1995/96 is comparable with the 20,130 deaths reported during this data year 2001/02 and the 21,991 deaths reported in 2000/01. Therefore any comparisons made in this chapter will be with the previous data year only.

Regional spread

Figure 10.1 shows the number of deaths reported by region as a percentage of the total. These regions are as they were at the time of data collection. Regions are now divided into four Regional Directorates of Health and Social Care and further divided by Strategic Health Authority.

Fig 10.1	Percentage of deaths by region			
Region	**2001/02 (%) n=20130**		**2000/01(%) n=20736**	
Eastern	1561	(7.8)	1764	(8.5)
London	2365	(11.7)	2718	(13.1)
North West	2711	(13.5)	2866	(13.8)
Northern & Yorkshire	2823	(14.0)	3004	(14.5)
South East	2849	(14.2)	2758	(13.3)
South West	2205	(11.0)	2147	(10.4)
Trent	1834	(9.1)	2077	(10.0)
West Midlands	1994	(9.9)	1723	(8.3)
Wales	1093	(5.4)	1017	(4.9)
Northern Ireland	436	(2.2)	399	(1.9)
Guernsey	22	(0.1)	22	(0.1)
Jersey	16	(0.1)	21	(0.1)
Isle of Man	31	(0.2)	26	(0.1)
Defence Secondary Care Agency	0	(0.0)	0	(0.0)
Independent	190	(0.9)	194	(0.9)

Exclusions

Of the 21,251 cases reported to NCEPOD, approximately 5% were excluded, the details of which are shown in Figure 10.2.

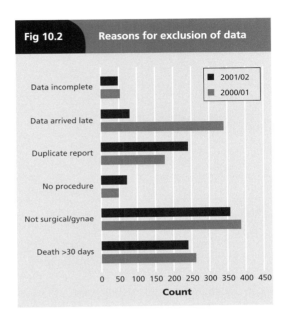

Fig 10.2 — **Reasons for exclusion of data**

Legend: ■ 2001/02 ■ 2000/01

Categories (top to bottom): Data incomplete, Data arrived late, Duplicate report, No procedure, Not surgical/gynae, Death >30 days

X-axis: Count (0, 50, 100, 150, 200, 250, 300, 350, 400, 450)

We are pleased to report that there is a marked decrease in the amount of data returned after the deadline of 31st September 2002. This is very encouraging as it is a 23% reduction on the amount of data returned late in the previous year.

Unfortunately no such improvement was seen in the amount of data returned incomplete despite an increase in clinical governance activity. This indicates that all information related to each patient is still not being recorded in their notes.

Prior to the 1999/00 collection year, NCEPOD noted an annual increase in the number of duplicate reports returned. This may have been associated with an increase in willingness to participate and local reporters ensuring that all data was reported to NCEPOD. However, in 1999/00 there was a marked decrease in the number of duplicates (but not in the overall data) indicating that data return was stabilising. However, each data collection year since has shown a small increase in the number of duplicates by approximately 2% per annum. This is also the case this year. This may represent the change in local reporters and it will be interesting to see how this changes in the future; with new data being submitted electronically we would expect to see a decline in duplication.

There has been no change in the proportion of procedures reported to us where death has occurred more than thirty days following a surgical procedure. We assume that such cases are sent to us simply because local reporters are wary about under reporting. It is important to note here that such cases are not excluded from the 2002/03 data collection year. From 1st April 2002 all deaths are reported to NCEPOD, regardless of whether or not a surgical procedure was performed. This data set includes the last six procedures performed prior to death but independent of specialty e.g. procedures performed by physicians will be included which will overcome the issue of the number of cases reported to NCEPOD each year where the procedure was not performed by a surgeon or gynaecologist. This will be relevant for the 2002/03 NCEPOD study as the data will be sampled for all patients that have died within 30 days of a therapeutic endoscopy regardless of the operator specialty. Interestingly, of the deaths excluded from the data set represented in this report because the patient was under the care of a physician, 65% were following an endoscopic procedure. The increased remit also overcomes the issue of the number of cases reported to NCEPOD each year where no procedure was performed.

As with previous years, we also have a number of cases, too small to warrant a group of their own, that falls into 'other'. This mainly includes data that is incorrect but also deaths at home, of which there was one, and deaths in the community of which there were two, although as of 1st April 2002, NCEPOD will also collect data from primary care Trusts as we extend our remit into primary care. The two cases of most concern were the two patients who had not in fact died.

Time between death and data return to NCEPOD

It is disappointing to note from Figure 10.3 that the time in which it takes for data to be returned to NCEPOD appears to be increasing. More deaths were reported after four months and the majority of data was returned more than six months late. There are a number of hospitals that do report in a very timely manner and we very much appreciate this. Late return of data can have a large impact on our studies as it becomes much harder for associated patient notes to be traced and makes it harder for clinicians to complete the questionnaires. It can also mean that a sudden flurry of questionnaires is sent to clinicians resulting in a bulk workload for them instead of receiving the questionnaires at more staggered intervals. We are aware however that often the data is late as it is has not been made available to the local reporter.

Age at death

Of the 20,130 cases included in this data set there seems to be little change in the mean age at which patients died compared with the previous year; this can be seen in Figure 10.4

It can be seen from Figure 10.4 that females have been operated on and subsequently died at an older age. The median age between females and males differs by approximately five years (79 v 75 in 2001 and 80 v 75 in 2000) and this is supported by the fact that females live to an older age in the general population [29]. This also suggests that the data reported to NCEPOD on an annual basis is consistent.

Time between surgery and death

It can be seen from Figure 10.5 that, consistent with the previous year, patients most commonly die within the first five days following surgery.

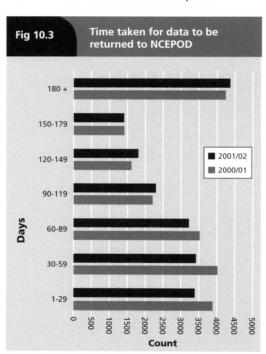

Fig 10.3 Time taken for data to be returned to NCEPOD

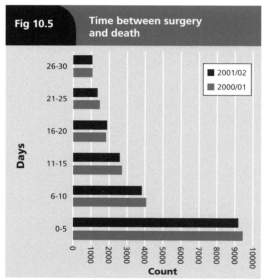

Fig 10.5 Time between surgery and death

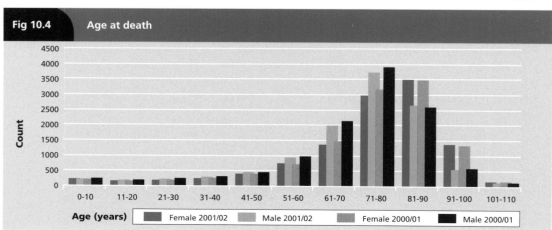

Fig 10.4 Age at death

REFERENCES

1. *Step guide to improving theatre performance.* NHS Modernisation Agency. London, 2002. **www.modern.nhs.uk**

2. *Operating theatres – Review of national findings.* Audit Commission. London, 2003. **www.audit-commission.gov.uk**

3. *Who Operates When?* A report by the National Confidential Enquiry into Perioperative Deaths 1995/96. London, 1997. **www.ncepod.org.uk**

4. *Trust Clusters 2002 – 2003.* Department of Health. **www.doh.gov.uk/ nhsperformanceindicators**

5. *Provision of Acute Hospital Services Consultation Document.* British Medical Association, The Royal College of Physicians of London, The Royal College of Surgeons of England. London, 1998. **www.bma.org.uk**

6. *The Provision of Emergency Surgical Services – An Organisational Framework.* The Royal College of Surgeons of England. London, 1997. **www.rcseng.ac.uk**

7. *The Report of the National Confidential Enquiry into Perioperative Deaths 1990.* NCEPOD. London, 1992. **www.ncepod.org.uk**

8. *CPR Guidance for clinical practice and training in hospitals..* The Resusciatation Council (UK). London, 2000. **www.resus.org.uk**

9. *Recommendations for Standards of Monitoring During Anaesthesia and Recovery.* The Association of Anaesthetists of Great Britain and Ireland. London, 2000. **www.aagbi.org.uk**

10. *Workforce Statistics, Medical and dental workforce census 1996 and 2001.* Department of Health. **www.doh.gov.uk/public/work_workforce**

11. Gaba DM, Howard SK. *Fatigue among clinicians and the safety of patients.* N Engl J Med 2002; **347 (16):** 1249-55.

12. Jha AK, Duncan BW, Bates DW. *Fatigue, sleepiness and medical error.* In: Shojania KG, Duncan BW, McDonald KM, Wachter RM eds. *Making health care safer: a critical analysis of patient safety practices.* Evidence report/ technology assessment no.43. Rockville Md. Agency for Healthcare Research and Quality, 2001: 519-31.

13. Howard SK, Rosekind MR, Katz JD, Berry AJ. *Fatigue in anesthesia: Implication and strategies for patient and provider safety.* Anesthesiology 2002 **97(5)**:1281-94.

14. Owens JA. *Sleep loss and fatigue in medical training.* Curr Opin Pulm Med 2001; **7**: 411-8.

15. Weinger MB, Ancoli-Israel S. *Sleep-deprivation and clinical performance.* JAMA 2002; **287**: 955-7.

16. *Day Surgery Follow-up.* Audt Commission. London, 1998. **www.audit-commission.gov.uk**

17. *A Short Cut to Better Services.* Audit Commission. London, 1990. **www.audit-commission.gov.uk**

18. *Guidelines for Day Case Surgery. Commission of the Provision of Surgical Services.* Royal College of Surgeons of England. London, 1992. **www.rcseng.ac.uk**

19. *Guidance for the Provision of Anaesthetic Services.* Royal College of Anaesthetists. London, 1999. **www.rcoa.ac.uk**

20. *Changing the way we operate.* The 2001 Report of the National Confidential Enquiry into Perioperative Deaths. NCEPOD. London, 2001. **www.ncepod.org.uk**

21. Kmietowicz K. *Some operating theatres are used only eight hours a week.* Brit Med J 2003; **326:** 1349.

22. *Fractured Neck of femur. Prevention &
    Management. Summary & recommendations of a
    report of the RCP.* J R Coll Physicians Lond
    1989 1-12.

23. *Prevention and management of hip
    fracture in older people. A national clinical
    guideline.* SIGN publication No 55,2002.
    www.show.scot.nhs.uk/SIGN

24. *Agenda AGM Appendix V.* Association of
    Surgeons of Great Britain and Ireland. May
    2003. **www.asgbi.org.uk**

25. Cook E. *The life of Florence Nightingale.*
    Macmillan. London, 1913.

26. *Good Medical Practice (para 12).* General
    Medical Council. London, 2001.
    www.gmc-uk.org

27. *A First Class Service: Quality in the new NHS.*
    Department of Health, 1998. **www.doh.gov.uk**

28. *National Minimum Standards Regulations,
    Independent Health Care.* Department of Health.
    London, 2002. **www.doh.gov.uk**

29. *Census 2001. National report for England
    and Wales.* Office National Statistics.
    www.statistics.gov.uk/STATBASE

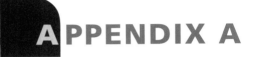

APPENDIX A

The following tables display the number of deaths reported to NCEPOD between April 1st 2001 to March 31st 2002 compared with the deaths reported between April 1st 2000 and March 31st 2001. All deaths occurred in hospitals within 30 days of a surgical procedure performed by a surgeon or gynaecologist.

ENGLAND

	2001/02	2000/01
Addenbrooke's NHS Trust	12	24
Aintree Hospitals NHS Trust	117	141
Airedale NHS Trust	57	1
Ashford & St Peter's Hospital NHS Trust	84	79
Barking, Havering and Redbridge Hospitals NHS Trust	216	235
Barnet and Chase Farm Hospitals NHS Trust	30	108
Barnsley District General Hospital NHS Trust	132	121
Barts and The London NHS Trust	183	191
Basildon & Thurrock General Hospitals NHS Trust	54	45
Bedford Hospital NHS Trust	44	119
Birmingham Children's Hospital NHS Trust	16	18
Birmingham Heartlands & Solihull NHS Trust	283	252
Birmingham Women's Healthcare NHS Trust	2	3
Blackburn, Hyndburn & Ribble Valley Healthcare NHS Trust	78	57
Blackpool, Fylde and Wyre Hospitals NHS Trust	272	300
Bolton Hospitals NHS Trust	77	129
Bradford Hospitals NHS Trust	127	194
Brighton and Sussex Hospitals NHS Trust	220	198
Bromley Hospitals NHS Trust	44	80
Burnley Health Care NHS Trust	96	1
Burton Hospitals NHS Trust	101	12
Calderdale & Huddersfield NHS Trust	148	140
Cardiothoracic Centre Liverpool NHS Trust (The)	43	62

	2001/02	2000/01
Central Manchester & Manchester Children's University Hospitals NHS Trust	59	74
Chelsea & Westminster Healthcare NHS Trust	31	15
Chesterfield & North Derbyshire Royal Hospital NHS Trust	46	62
Christie Hospital NHS Trust	2	3
City Hospitals Sunderland NHS Trust	174	207
Countess of Chester Hospital NHS Trust	117	131
Dartford & Gravesham NHS Trust	110	65
Doncaster and Bassetlaw Hospitals NHS Trust	120	156
Dudley Group of Hospitals NHS Trust (The)	135	125
Ealing Hospital NHS Trust	No deaths reported	8
East & North Hertfordshire NHS Trust	77	18
East Cheshire NHS Trust	26	31
East Kent Hospitals NHS Trust	226	312
East Somerset NHS Trust	57	26
East Sussex Hospitals NHS Trust	123	158
Epsom and St Helier NHS Trust	112	116
Essex Rivers Healthcare NHS Trust	138	143
Frimley Park Hospitals NHS Trust	98	64
Gateshead Health NHS Trust	74	77
George Eliot Hospital NHS Trust	63	67
Gloucestershire Hospitals NHS Trust	300	398
Good Hope Hospital NHS Trust	81	84
Great Ormond Street Hospital for Children NHS Trust (The)	28	36
Guy's & St Thomas' Hospital Trust	41	79
Hammersmith Hospitals NHS Trust	158	148
Harrogate Healthcare NHS Trust	71	89
Heatherwood and Wexham Park Hospitals NHS Trust	112	143
Hereford Hospitals NHS Trust	26	12
Hillingdon Hospital NHS Trust	41	30
Hinchingbrooke Health Care NHS Trust	45	61
Homerton Univeristy Hospital NHS Trust	30	33
Hull and East Yorkshire Hospitals NHS Trust	233	177
Ipswich Hospital NHS Trust	233	148
Isle of Wight Healthcare NHS Trust	75	74
James Paget Healthcare NHS Trust	133	101
Kettering General Hospital NHS Trust	77	114
King's College Hospital NHS Trust	102	134
King's Lynn & Wisbech Hospitals NHS Trust	50	91
Kingston Hospital NHS Trust	90	17
Lancashire Teaching Hospitals NHS Trust	147	155
Leeds Teaching Hospitals NHS Trust (The)	371	517
Lewisham Hospital NHS Trust (The)	67	116

	2001/02	2000/01
Liverpool Women's Hospital NHS Trust	5	4
Luton and Dunstable Hospital NHS Trust	79	50
Maidstone and Tunbridge Wells NHS Trust	66	207
Mayday Health Care NHS Trust	77	60
Medway NHS Trust	139	134
Mid Cheshire Hospitals NHS Trust	154	164
Mid-Essex Hospital Services NHS Trust	93	94
Mid Staffordshire General Hospitals NHS Trust	52	77
Mid Yorkshire Hospitals NHS Trust	226	217
Milton Keynes General NHS Trust	26	30
Moorfields Eye Hospital NHS Trust	0	0
Morecambe Bay Hospitals NHS Trust	146	119
Newcastle upon Tyne Hospitals NHS Trust (The)	418	440
Newham Healthcare NHS Trust	36	41
Norfolk & Norwich University Hospital NHS Trust	187	264
North Bristol NHS Trust	161	179
North Cheshire Hospitals NHS Trust	26	39
North Cumbria Acute Hospitals NHS Trust	63	73
North Durham Healthcare NHS Trust	98	58
North Hampshire Hospitals NHS Trust	69	56
North Middlesex University Hospital NHS Trust	94	93
North Staffordshire Hospital NHS Trust	96	79
North Tees and Hartlepool NHS Trust	122	99
North West London Hospitals NHS Trust	126	127
Northampton General Hospital NHS Trust	104	65
Northern Devon Healthcare NHS Trust	48	64
Northern Lincolnshire & Goole Hospitals Trust	179	83
Northumbria Healthcare NHS Trust	172	144
Nottingham City Hospital NHS Trust	37	75
Nuffield Orthopaedic Centre NHS Trust	8	6
Oxford Radcliffe Hospital NHS Trust	269	269
Papworth Hospital NHS Trust	89	107
Pennine Acute Hospitals NHS Trust (The)	274	239
Peterborough Hospitals NHS Trust	109	134
Plymouth Hospitals NHS Trust	320	326
Poole Hospital NHS Trust	140	152
Portsmouth Hospitals NHS Trust	110	114
Princess Alexandra Hospital NHS Trust (The)	1	3
Princess Royal Hospital NHS Trust (The)	32	11
Queen Elizabeth Hospital NHS Trust	69	67
Queen Mary's Sidcup NHS Trust	10	2
Queen Victoria Hospital NHS Trust (The)	5	16

APPENDICES

	2001/02	2000/01
Queen's Medical Centre Nottingham University Hospital NHS Trust	253	326
Robert Jones/Agnes Hunt Orthopaedic Hospital NHS Trust	1	2
Rotherham General Hospitals NHS Trust	129	132
Royal Berkshire & Battle Hospitals NHS Trust	22	22
Royal Bournemouth & Christchurch Hospitals NHS Trust	67	96
Royal Brompton & Harefield NHS Trust	119	137
Royal Cornwall Hospitals Trust	240	224
Royal Devon & Exeter Healthcare NHS Trust	233	267
Royal Free Hampstead NHS Trust	2	128
Royal Liverpool & Broadgreen University Hospitals NHS Trust	127	221
Royal Liverpool Children's NHS Trust (The)	19	22
Royal Marsden Trust (The)	31	27
Royal National Orthopaedic Hospital NHS Trust	3	10
Royal Orthopaedic Hospital NHS Trust (The)	9	5
Royal Shrewsbury Hospitals NHS Trust	31	22
Royal Surrey County Hospital NHS Trust	63	38
Royal United Hospital Bath NHS Trust	31	3
Royal West Sussex Trust (The)	62	68
Royal Wolverhampton Hospitals NHS Trust (The)	137	136
Salford Royal Hospitals NHS Trust	160	156
Salisbury Health Care NHS Trust	45	40
Sandwell & West Birmingham Hospitals NHS Trust	157	218
Scarborough & North East Yorkshire Health Care NHS Trust	113	101
Sheffield Children's Hospital NHS Trust	3	15
Sheffield Teaching Hospitals NHS Trust	318	364
Sherwood Forest Hospitals NHS Trust	110	117
South Buckinghamshire NHS Trust	79	47
South Devon Healthcare NHS Trust	133	58
South Durham Healthcare NHS Trust	81	71
South Manchester University Hospitals NHS Trust	80	95
South Tees Hospitals NHS Trust	212	248
South Tyneside Healthcare Trust	41	54
South Warwickshire General Hospitals NHS Trust	76	79
Southampton University Hospitals NHS Trust	273	282
Southend Hospital NHS Trust	85	116
Southern Derbyshire Acute Hospitals NHS Trust	116	129
Southport & Ormskirk Hospitals NHS Trust	72	114
St George's Healthcare NHS Trust	250	289
St Helens and Knowsley Hospitals NHS Trust	124	131
St Mary's NHS Trust	77	40
Stockport NHS Trust	85	74
Stoke Mandeville Hospital NHS Trust	48	42

	2001/02	2000/01
Surrey & Sussex Healthcare NHS Trust	139	No deaths reported
Swindon & Marlborough NHS Trust	90	93
Tameside and Glossop Acute Services NHS Trust	64	50
Taunton & Somerset NHS Trust	16	24
Trafford Healthcare NHS Trust	26	24
United Bristol Healthcare NHS Trust	166	72
United Lincolnshire Hospitals NHS Trust	223	218
University College London Hospitals NHS Trust	147	160
University Hospital Birmingham NHS Trust	194	182
University Hospitals Coventry and Warwickshire NHS Trust	235	133
University Hospitals of Leicester NHS Trust	168	279
Walsall Hospitals NHS Trust	104	111
Walton Centre for Neurology & Neurosurgery NHS Trust	23	26
West Dorset General Hospitals NHS Trust	111	71
West Hertfordshire Hospitals NHS Trust	124	152
West Middlesex University Hospital NHS Trust	32	34
West Suffolk Hospitals NHS Trust	103	94
Weston Area Health Trust	48	54
Whipps Cross University Hospital NHS Trust	70	112
Whittington Hospital NHS Trust	51	45
Winchester & Eastleigh Healthcare NHS Trust	72	27
Wirral Hospital NHS Trust	158	175
Worcestershire Acute Hospitals	168	95
Worthing & Southlands Hospitals NHS Trust	182	128
Wrightington, Wigan & Leigh NHS Trust	142	129
York Health Services NHS Trust	86	97

WALES

	2001/02	2000/01
Bro Morgannwg NHS Trust	10	7
Cardiff and Vale NHS Trust	29	352
Carmarthenshire NHS Trust	72	90
Ceredigion & Mid Wales NHS Trust	28	27
Conwy & Denbighshire NHS Trust	89	60
Gwent Healthcare NHS Trust	230	222
North East Wales NHS Trust	59	93
North Glamorgan NHS Trust	46	33
North West Wales NHS Trust	87	60
Pembrokeshire & Derwen NHS Trust	43	43
Pontypridd & Rhondda NHS Trust	76	62
Swansea NHS Trust	80	218

NORTHERN IRELAND

	2001/02	2000/01
Altnagelvin Hospitals Health & Social Services Trust	20	12
Belfast City Hospital Health & Social Services Trust	56	58
Causeway Health & Social Services Trust	7	11
Craigavon Area Hospital Group Trust	30	43
Down Lisburn Health & Social Services Trust	25	23
Green Park Healthcare Trust	6	4
Mater Hospital Belfast Health & Social Services Trust	25	30
Newry & Mourne Health & Social Services Trust	26	30
Royal Group of Hospitals & Dental Hospitals & Maternity Hospitals Trust	119	106
Sperrin Lakeland Health & Social Care NHS Trust	19	9
Ulster Community & Hospitals NHS Trust	91	55
United Hospitals Health & Social Services Trust	12	18

INDEPENDENT

	2001/02	2000/01
Abbey Hospitals	0	*
Aspen Healthcare	3	2
Benenden Hospital Trust (The)	0	0
BMI Healthcare	65	78
BUPA	35	31
Capio Health Care UK	9	12
HCA International	52	37
King Edward VII Hospital	3	3
King Edward VII's Hospital Sister Agnes	2	2
London Clinic (The)	7	13
Nuffield Hospitals	9	16
St Anthony's Hospital	4	*
St Joseph's Hospital	1	*

* Did not commence participation in Enquiry until April 2001.

OTHER HOSPITALS

	2001/02	2000/01
DSCA - the Princess Mary's Hospital, Akrotiri, Cyprus	0	No deaths reported
Isle of Man Department of Health & Social Security	31	26
States of Guernsey Board of Health	22	22
States of Jersey Health & Social Services	16	21

APPENDICES

APPENDIX B

GLOSSARY

American Society of Anesthesiologists (ASA) classification of physical status

ASA 1:   A normal healthy patient.

ASA 2:   A patient with mild systemic disease.

ASA 3:   A patient with severe systemic disease.

ASA 4:   A patient with severe systemic disease that is a constant threat to life.

ASA 5:   A moribund patient who is not expected to survive without the operation.

ASA 6:   A declared brain-dead patient whose organs are being removed for donor purposes.

Classification of operation (NCEPOD definition)

EMERGENCY: Immediate life-saving operation, resuscitation, simultaneous with surgical treatment (e.g. trauma, ruptured aortic aneurysm). Operation usually within one hour.

URGENT: Operation as soon as possible after resuscitation (e.g. irreducible hernia, intussusception, oesophageal atresia, intestinal obstruction, major fractures). Operation within 24 hours.

SCHEDULED: An early operation but not immediately life-saving (e.g. malignancy). Operation usually within three weeks.

ELECTIVE: Operation at a time to suit both patient and surgeon (e.g. cholecystectomy, joint replacement).

Periods of time

DAY: 08:00 to 17:59

EVENING: 18:00 to 23:59

NIGHT: 00:00 to 07:59

OUT OF HOURS: 18:00 to 17:59 Monday to Friday and all day Saturday and Sunday

OFFICE HOURS: 08:00 to 17:59 Monday to Friday

NCEPOD list

Dedicated emergency or trauma list which is staffed for emergency cases.

APPENDICES

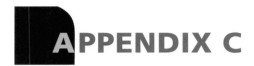

APPENDIX C

ABBREVIATIONS

A&E	Accident & Emergency
AAA	Abdominal Aortic Aneurysm
ASA	American Society of Anesthesiologists
BMA	British Medical Association
CHI	Commission for Health Improvement
DoH	Department of Health
ECG	Electrocardiogram
HES	Hospital Episode Statistics
MRI	Magnetic Resonance Imaging
NHS	National Health Service
NICE	National Institute for Clinical Excellence
OPCS	Office of Population, Census and Surveys
PAS	Patient Administration System
SAC	Specialist Advisory Committee
SAS	Staff grade and Associate Specialists
SASM	Scottish Audit of Surgical Mortality
SHO 1,2	Senior House Officer, year 1 or 2
SpR 1,2,3,4	Specialist Registrar, year 1, 2, 3 or 4
WOW I	Who Operates When? (Published in 1997)
WOW II	Who Operates When? II (This report)
#	Fracture

APPENDIX D

WHO OPERATES WHEN? II SURGICAL OPERATIONS ENQUIRY 2002

NOTES ON COMPLETION OF THE QUESTIONNAIRE INCLUDING DEFINITIONS

GENERAL

Please complete the questionnaire (or include the data in a print-out from your computer system) for every *theatre case* or *operative procedure* within an *operating theatre* performed by a surgeon, gynaecologist or dental surgeon in the 7-day period specified by NCEPOD.

Theatre case - One visit of a patient to an operating theatre to undergo one or more operative procedures.

Operating theatre - A room in a hospital containing one or more operating tables or other similar devices. An operating theatre accommodates one or two patients at a time during and only during the period in which, under the direct supervision of a medical or dental practitioner, the patient can undergo operative treatment for the prevention, cure, relief or diagnosis of disease.

Included:
- All main, fully equipped, operating theatres and day case theatres
- Fully equipped operating theatre in an A&E department

Excluded:
- Dental treatment room or surgery containing a dental chair
- X-ray room whether diagnostic or therapeutic
- Obstetric delivery room or theatres
- Endoscopy rooms
- A & E treatment rooms

Operative procedure – **Any procedure carried out by a surgeon or gynaecologist with or without an anaesthetist, involving local, regional or general anaesthesia or sedation.**

All of the data will remain confidential at the NCEPOD office and will be destroyed once the report has been published (Autumn 2003). It is particularly important to note that the collection of clinicians' names is for administrative purposes only and all such data will be kept confidential within the NCEPOD offices. We will be writing to consultant surgeons and anaesthetists about some of the cases.

THE FORM WILL BE ELECTRONICALLY SCANNED. USE A BLACK OR BLUE PEN – DO <u>NOT</u> USE A RED PEN. PLEASE COMPLETE ALL QUESTIONS WITH EITHER PRINTED CAPITALS OR A BOLD CROSS. IF YOU MAKE A MISTAKE PLEASE 'BLACK OUT' THE WHOLE BOX AND MARK THE CORRECT ONE.

APPENDICES

Q1. *Hospital number* - this is to enable us to have a unique identifier – combined with the date of procedure – for each theatre case that we will analyse. It is not necessary for us to have the name of the patient.

Q2. No question guidance.

Q3. *Sex* - male, female or indeterminate.

Q4. *Date of admission* – The date on which the patient was admitted to the hospital (i.e. on the same site) in which the procedure was performed.

Q5. *Admission type:*

Inpatient – patients admitted with a planned stay overnight either as an emergency or as an elective case.

Day case – a surgical day case is a patient who is admitted for investigations or operation on a planned non-resident basis (i.e. no overnight stay).

Q6. No question guidance.

Q7. *ASA status* – Please enter 1-6 as appropriate

1 – A normal healthy patient.
2 – A patient with mild systemic disease.
3 – A patient with severe systemic disease.
4 – A patient with severe systemic disease that is a constant threat to life.
5 – A moribund patient who is not expected to survive without the operation.
6 – A declared brain-dead patient whose organs are being removed for donor purposes.

Q8. *Theatre session type:* Theatre cases are classified by whether the visit to the operating theatre occurred within a scheduled session or in an unscheduled session.

A theatre case is considered *'scheduled'* if it was carried out during a period of time allocated to a scheduled operating theatre session and by a member of a consultant firm of the same specialty as that allocated to the session. If the theatre case is part of a scheduled session that has overrun it should still be classified as 'scheduled' regardless of the time of the case.

A theatre case is **'unscheduled'** if it is not within a scheduled session or is carried out by a member of a consultant firm not allocated to that particular scheduled session.

'Emergency surgical' and **'Emergency trauma'** session types are those sessions that are allocated to a consultant on a regular basis for patients whose visit to the operating theatre was not foreseen but takes place as a result of accident or illness. These sessions are fully staffed.

Q9. *Classification of theatre case:*

Emergency: Immediate life-saving operation, resuscitation simultaneous with surgical treatment (e.g. trauma, ruptured aortic aneurysm). Operation usually within one hour.

Urgent: Operation as soon as possible after resuscitation (e.g. irreducible hernia, major fracture). Operation usually within 24 hours.
Scheduled: Early operation but not immediately life-saving (e.g. malignancy). Operation usually within three weeks.
Elective: Operation at a time to suit both patient and surgeon (e.g. cholecystectomy, joint replacement) resource permitting.

Q10. No question guidance.

Q11. **Start time of anaesthesia** – the start of the anaesthesia where this takes place either in the operating theatre or in the anaesthetic room. Leave blank if no anaesthetic is given.

Q12. **Start time of surgery** – the start of procedure regardless of whether an anaesthetic is given. This should be 'knife to skin'.

Q13. No question guidance.

Q14. **Indication for operation/surgical diagnosis** - the reason for the operation.

Q15. **Procedure(s) performed** – please provide the name(s) of the procedure.

Q16. **Name of senior surgeon present** – this should be the name of the most senior surgeon actually in the operating theatre – scrubbed or unscrubbed.

Q17. **Grade of senior surgeon present:**

CON	Consultant
ASS	Associate Specialist
SGR	Staff Grade/Trust Doctor
CLA	Clinical Assistant/ Hospital Practitioner
SPC	SpR with CCST
SSF	Sub-specialty fellow
SP4	SpR year 4 or greater
SP3	SpR year 3
SP2	SpR year 2
SP1	SpR year 1
SPV	Visiting SpR
PSH	Premier Senior House Officer (or SHO for >2 years)
SH2	SHO year 2
SH1	SHO year 1
PHO	Pre-registration House Officer
OTH	Other

+

NATIONAL CEPOD

WHO OPERATES WHEN II

This form will be electronically scanned. Please use a black pen. Please complete all questions with either printed capitals or a bold cross. If you make a mistake, please "black-out" the box and re-enter the correct information.

Section One - The patient

1. Hospital no. of patient

2. Year of birth

3. Sex
M   F   I

4. Date of admission
d d   m m   y y

5. Admission type
(please tick only one)
☐ In patient – elective   ☐ In patient - emergency   ☐ Day case

6. Date of procedure
d d   m m   y y

7. ASA Status ☐ (1 to 6)
(Note: We do not use the E sub-classification)

+

Section Two – The theatre session

8. Theatre session type
(please tick only one)
☐ Scheduled
☐ Emergency surgical
☐ Emergency trauma
☐ Unscheduled

9. Classification of theatre case
(please tick only one)
☐ Emergency
☐ Urgent
☐ Scheduled
☐ Elective

10. Location of procedure
(please tick only one)
☐ Theatre suite
☐ Day case unit
☐ Other (please specify)

Section Three – The procedure

11. Start time of anaesthesia   (please use the 24 hour clock, 00:00 to 23:59)

12. Start time of surgery   (please use the 24 hour clock, 00:00 to 23:59)

13. Type(s) of anaesthetic
(may be multiple)
☐ a. Local
☐ d. General
☐ b. Epidural/Spinal
☐ e. Sedation
☐ c. Other regional

14. Indication for operation /
surgical diagnosis

15. Procedure(s) performed

Section Four – The surgeon

16. Name of most senior surgeon
present during procedure

Mr / Mrs / Miss / Ms / Dr / Prof   (please ring)   **Initials**

Surname

17. Grade of most senior surgeon
present during procedure
(see attached information sheet for three digit codes)

+   +

APPENDICES

Q18/ No question guidance.
Q20.

Q21. **Out of hours** – 18:01 to 07:59 Monday to Friday and all hours on a Saturday, Sunday or Bank Holiday.

Q22. **Name of consultant surgeon** – this should always be the name of a consultant surgeon or gynaecologist in charge of the team performing the operation.

Q23. **Specialty of consultant surgeon:**

GEN	General
A&E	Accident & Emergency
CAR	Cardiac/Thoracic/Cardiothoracic
O&G	Obstetrics/Gynaecology
NEU	Neurosurgery
OPH	Ophthalmology
MAX	Oral & Maxillofacial
ORT	Orthopaedic & Trauma
ENT	Otorhinolaryngology
PAE	Paediatric
PLA	Plastic
TRA	Transplantation
URO	Urology
VAS	Vascular
OTH	Other

Q24. **Name of senior anaesthetist present** – please note that this will not always be the anaesthetist at the beginning of the procedure. If a more senior anaesthetist goes into the theatre, his or her details should be recorded.

If no anaesthetist was present at all (e.g. local anaesthetic by surgeon only) please enter "LOCAL" into the surname box.

Q25. **Grade of senior anaesthetist.** See definitions for Q17.

Q26/ No question guidance.
Q27.

Q28. **Out of hours.** See definitions for Q21.

Q29. **Duty, on-call or responsible consultant** – if the most senior anaesthetist was <u>not</u> a consultant, please provide the name of the consultant who is nominally responsible for the operating list <u>or</u> the name of the consultant who was on-call at the time of the operation. If this information is not available, please write 'N/A'.

Q30. **Level of supervision provided** – by the consultant named in Q29. These are RCA definitions.
Immediately available – supervisor is actually with the trainee or can be within seconds of being called.
Local supervision – supervisor on same geographical site, is immediately available for advice and is able to be with the trainee within 10 minutes of being called.
Distant supervision – supervisor is rapidly available for advice but is off the hospital site and/or separated from the trainee by over 10 minutes.

Q31. **Time out of theatre** – the time a theatre case leaves the operating theatre, <u>not</u> the time of leaving the theatre suite.

Q32. This question is to explore whether theatre staff are doubling up as recovery staff thus limiting throughput in theatres.

Q33/ No question guidance.
Q34.

18. Was the senior surgeon present a locum? ☐ Y ☐ N

19. Years in grade of senior surgeon present ☐

20. If senior surgeon present is a trainee, is he/she working (please tick only one)
   ☐ An on-call rota - If on a rota, please specify - 1 in ☐ days
   ☐ A full shift
   ☐ A partial shift

21. If senior surgeon is a consultant and the procedure was commenced out of hours
   a. Was the surgeon on call? ☐ Y ☐ N
   b. Will the surgeon have time off **following** out-of-hours duties? ☐ Y ☐ N

22. If senior surgeon present is not a consultant, please state name of **consultant surgeon** in charge of patient
   Mr / Mrs / Miss / Ms / Dr / Prof (please ring)   Initials ☐☐
   Surname ☐☐☐☐☐☐☐☐☐☐☐☐☐☐☐☐☐☐
   NCEPOD use only ☐☐☐☐

23. Specialty of **consultant surgeon** in charge ☐ (see attached information sheet for three digit codes)

Section Five – The anaesthetist

24. Name of most senior anaesthetist **present** during the procedure
   Dr / Prof (please ring)   Initials ☐☐
   Surname ☐☐☐☐☐☐☐☐☐☐☐☐☐☐☐☐☐☐

25. Grade of most senior anaesthetist **present** during procedure ☐ (please see attached information sheet for three digit codes)

26. Years in grade of senior anaesthetist present ☐

27. If senior anaesthetist present is a trainee, is he/she working (please tick only one)
   ☐ An on-call rota - If on a rota, please specify - 1 in ☐ days
   ☐ A full shift
   ☐ A partial shift

28. If senior anaesthetist is a consultant and the procedure was commenced out of hours
   Will the anaesthetist have time off **following** out-of-hours duties? ☐ Y ☐ N

29. If senior anaesthetist present is not a consultant, please state name of duty, on–call or responsible **consultant**
   Dr / Prof (please ring)   Initials ☐☐
   Surname ☐☐☐☐☐☐☐☐☐☐☐☐☐☐☐☐☐☐
   NCEPOD use only ☐☐☐☐

30. If senior anaesthetist is not a consultant, was there
   ☐ Immediately available supervision   ☐ Local supervision   ☐ Distant supervision   (please tick only one)

Section Six – Recovery and final destination

31. Time patient out of theatre ☐☐ ☐☐ (please use the 24 hour clock, 00:00 to 23:59)

32. Would the arrangements for the recovery of this patient prevent the start of another case (if required)? ☐ Y ☐ N

33. Was the patient sent to recovery? ☐ Y ☐ N   33a. Length of stay in recovery ☐ hrs ☐ mins

34. Final destination after leaving suite (please tick only one)
   ☐ HDU
   ☐ ICU
   ☐ CCU
   ☐ Appropriate surgical specialty ward
   ☐ General surgical ward
   ☐ General medical ward
   ☐ Home
   ☐ Died in theatre
   ☐ Other (see 34a below)

34a. If "Other", please specify ☐☐☐☐☐☐☐☐☐☐☐☐☐☐☐☐☐☐☐☐☐☐☐☐☐☐

+

NATIONAL CEPOD

General data questionnaire for Who Operates When II

Hospital name

This form will be electronically scanned. Please use a black or blue pen. Please complete all questions with either printed capitals or a bold cross.   For example | 2 | 3 | 4 | 5 | 6 |

or   X (y)   □ (n)

If you make a mistake, please "black-out" the box and re-enter the correct information.   ■ (y)   X (n)

The hospital

1. How many surgical beds are there in this hospital? (all surgical specialties)   [ ][ ][ ][ ] 1

2. What was the number of elective admissions for the year 2000/2001?   [ ][ ][ ][ ][ ] 2

3. What was the number of emergency admissions for the year 2000/2001?   [ ][ ][ ][ ][ ] 3

Theatres

4. How many surgical theatres are there in the hospital?   [ ][ ][ ] 4

5. Are there daytime trauma theatre sessions i.e. where a theatre is staffed and set aside exclusively for emergency or urgent orthopaedic or trauma operations?   *(if no go to Q6)*   □ (y)   □ (n) 5

5a. If yes, how many trauma sessions are there each week?   [ ][ ][ ] 5a

6. Are there daytime emergency theatre sessions i.e. where a theatre is staffed and set aside exclusively for emergency or urgent operations (excluding the dedicated trauma lists above)?   *(if no go to Q7)*   □ (y)   □ (n) 6

6a. If yes, how many emergency sessions are there each week?   [ ][ ][ ] 6a

7. Are emergency out of hours operations undertaken in the main theatre complex?   □ (y)   □ (n) 7

+

Main theatre recovery

8. Is the recovery area available and staffed, by dedicated recovery
staff, 24 hours a day, 7 days a week?   *(if yes go to Q9)*   ☐ y   ☐ n   8

8a. If no, please enter the appropriate code in each of the 9 boxes
for who would normally recover patients out of hours

Time slot	Weekdays	Saturday	Sunday
18:00 – 22:00			
22:01 – 23:59			
00:00 – 07:59			

A - dedicated on-call recovery nurse   D - anaesthetist
B - on-call theatre staff   E - other (please specify below)
C - on-call operating department personnel

8b. ☐☐☐☐☐☐☐☐☐☐☐☐☐☐☐☐☐☐☐☐☐☐☐☐☐☐☐ 8b
☐☐☐☐☐☐☐☐☐☐☐☐☐☐☐☐☐☐☐☐☐☐☐☐☐☐☐

9. For each recovery bed/trolley space, is there a: a. Pulse oximeter   ☐ y   ☐ n   9a

b. ECG monitor   ☐ y   ☐ n   9b

10. Do the recovery staff undergo resuscitation training at least annually?   ☐ y   ☐ n   10

Management and audit

11. Is there a nominated arbitrator to decide clinical priorities in theatres?   ☐ y   ☐ n   11
                                                                (if no go to Q12)

11a. If yes does that person have   A - A nursing background   ☐ y

B - A medical background   ☐ y

C - A solely management background   ☐ y

12. Do the operating theatres have clinical audit meetings?   *(if no go to Q13)*   ☐ y   ☐ n   12

12a. If yes, is the pattern of work in the operating theatres regularly reviewed?   ☐ y   ☐ n

13. Does the information acquired by the operating theatres about the case
also record the grades of all anaesthetists and surgeons present?   ☐ y   ☐ n   13

OUT OF HOURS QUESTIONNAIRE

Dr A.N.Other

NCEPOD ID	Hospital, Hospital No. and senior surgeon/ anaesthetist	Date of procedure	Procedure performed	Reason procedure performed out of hours	Private patient? (tick if yes)
Nnnnnnn	Anywhere Hospital Nnnnnna A Person	dd-mmm-yy	Aaaaaaaaaaaaaa	(Free text for consultant to complete)	

A proforma as shown above was sent to consultant surgeons and anaesthetists where surgery had been undertaken out of hours. The consultant completed the 'Reason procedure performed out of hours' box and the 'Private patient' box.

APPENDIX E

NCEPOD CORPORATE STRUCTURE

The National Confidential Enquiry into Perioperative Deaths (NCEPOD) is an independent body to which a corporate commitment has been made by the associations, colleges and faculties related to its areas of activity. Each of these bodies nominates members of the steering group.

Steering Group
(as at 31 July 2003)

Members

Dr S Bridgman	(Faculty of Public Health Medicine)
Dr M Burke	(Royal College of Pathologists)
Professor I T Gilmore	(Royal College of Physicians)
Dr D Justins	(Royal College of Anaesthetists)
Mr B Keogh	(Royal College of Surgeons of England)
Mr G T Layer	(Association of Surgeons of Great Britain and Ireland)
Professor D M Luesley	(Royal College of Obstetricians and Gynaecologists)
Dr A Nicholson	(Royal College of Radiologists)
Dr P Nightingale	(Royal College of Anaesthetists)
Dr M Pearson	(Royal College of Physicians)
Mr B F Ribeiro	(Royal College of Surgeons)
Dr P J Simpson	(Royal College of Anaesthetists)
Mr L F A Stassen	(Faculty of Dental Surgery, Royal College of Surgeons of England)
Mr M F Sullivan	(Royal College of Surgeons of England)
Professor T Treasure	(Royal College of Surgeons of England)
Dr D Whitaker	(Association of Anaesthetists of Great Britain and Ireland)
Mrs M Wishart	(Royal College of Opthalmologists)

APPENDICES

Observers

Mrs M Ibbetson (Lay representative)

Dr P A Knapman (Coroners' Society of England and Wales)

Professor P Littlejohns (National Institute for Clinical Excellence)

Ms M McElligott (Royal College of Nursing)

Mr P Milligan (Institute of Healthcare Management)

NCEPOD is a company, limited by guarantee and a registered charity, managed by trustees.

Trustees

Dr P J Simpson (Chairman)

Mr M F Sullivan (Treasurer)

Mr G T Layer

Professor T Treasure

Clinical co-ordinators

The trustees (on behalf of the steering group) appoint the lead clinical co-ordinator for a defined tenure. The lead clinical co-ordinator leads the review of the data relating to the annual sample, advises the steering group and writes the reports. The trustees also appoint clinical co-ordinators again for a fixed tenure. All clinical co-ordinators must be engaged in active academic/clinical practice (in the NHS) during the full term of office.

Lead clinical co-ordinator

Dr A J G Gray

Clinical co-ordinators

Anaesthesia Dr D G Mason
Dr K M Sherry

Medicine Dr G P Findlay
Dr T D Wardle

Pathology Professor S B Lucas

Surgery Mr S R Carter
Mr M Lansdown
Mr I C Martin

Funding

The total annual cost of NCEPOD was approximately £616,000 in 2001/02. We are pleased to acknowledge the support of the following organisations, who contributed to funding the Enquiry in 2001/2002.

National Institute for Clinical Excellence

Welsh Office

Health and Social Services Executive (Northern Ireland)

States of Guernsey Board of Health

States of Jersey

Department of Health and Social Security, Isle of Man Government

Abbey Group

Aspen Healthcare

Benenden Hospital

BMI Healthcare

BUPA

Community Hospitals Group

Foscote Private Hospital

HCA International

Horder Centre for Arthritis

Hospital of St John & St Elizabeth

King Edward VII Hospital, Midhurst

King Edward VII's Hospital Sister Agnes

New Victoria Hospital

Nuffield Hospitals

St Anthony's (Cheam)

St Joseph's Hospital

The Heart Hospital

The London Clinic

This funding covers the total cost of the Enquiry, including administrative salaries and re-imbursements for clinical co-ordinators, office accommodation charges, computer and other equipment as well as travelling expenses for the clinical co-ordinators, steering group and advisory groups.

APPENDIX F

LOCAL REPORTERS

Listed below are the contacts who co-ordinated the collection of the Who Operates When? II data, and reported deaths to NCEPOD between April 2001 and March 2002.

Abbott D.
Abdelrahman J.
Abdulla A.K.
Abramczuk K.
Ahmed K.
Alborough E.
Aldred V.
Al-Jafari M.S.
Allen J.
Allinson F.
Allinson S.
Allum S.
Anand K.
Anderson F.
Armitage D.
Arnold M.
Arrowsmith L.
Arthur P.
Asher S.
Ashfield P.
Ashpole E.
Aspinall J.
Atherton M.
Attanoos R.
Attenborough J.
Aucott C.
Austin A.
Avery P.
Bailey A.
Bairstow J.
Baker P.
Balmforth R.
Bane M.
Barber P.
Barker J.
Barlow J.
Barnes D.
Barrett S.
Bartlett J.
Barwick L.
Beach D.
Beaty J.
Beaver A.
Beck G.
Bell M.
Bell S.
Bellamy P.

Benbow E.W.
Bentley J.
Beresford P.
Beresford-Huey J.
Berresford P.A.
Berry J.
Berry J.
Beswick K.
Bibby C.
Biddle E.
Bidmead J.
Biffin A.H.
Blackburn M.
Blackley S.
Blewitt R.W.
Boakes C.
Bostock K.
Bowman L.
Boyd T.
Bradbury H.
Bradgate M.
Bradshaw J.
Brady H.
Brasier H.
Brassington S.
Breakell L.
Bridgeman N.
Bridgwater R.
Britchford G.
Britt D.
Broddle A.
Broome J.
Broomhall J.
Brown A.
Brown R.
Brown S.A.
Brown S.
Browne B.
Brundler M.A.
Brunt A.
Bullock C.
Burchett K.
Burdge A.H.
Burdock F.
Burgoyner J.
Butler R.
Calder C.

Caley K.	Cose S.	El-Jabbour J.	Goodwin C.
Calleja M.	Coyne J.	Elliott K.	Gordon F.
Cameron C.	Craddock E.	Ellyatt J.	Gotting A.
Camp A.V.	Cranley B.	Ely P.	Goulding S.
Camp A.V.	Crawford M.	Enstone P.	Graham Y.
Campbell M.	Crawshaw B.	Evans C.	Gray A.J.G.
Capstick D.	Crissell T.	Evans G.	Gray L.
Carlisle R.	Critchley G.	Evans J.	Greaves M.
Carr C.	Cross S.	Evans J.E.	Green S.
Carty D.	Crossley J.	Everitt J.	Greener C.
Casey S.	Crossley P.	Falconer M.	Greenwood S.
Caslin A.W.	Crowther P.	Farrell D.	Grunwald C.
Cassidy J.	Crozier J.	Fattah A.	Gunn S.
Castleton B.	Cubbon K.	Fear J.	Gurney L.
Cater M.	Curran S.	Fernandez C.	Hackett R.
Cathcart W.	Curtis B.	Fernwick L.	Hadley T.
Chambers J.	Cutts M.W.J.	Finch J.	Haffenden M.
Chan D.	Da Silva S.	Flanagan D.	Halfacre J.
Choudhury S.	Damant M.	Flett A.	Hall H.
Clark A.	Damarell-Kewell S.	Flynn P.J.	Hall M.T.
Clarke N.	Daniel L.	Ford J.	Hallam D.
Clarke S.	Danko S.	Ford L.	Hamilton I.
Claw R.	Davies D.	Forni J.	Hamilton J.N.
Clegg L.	Davies J.	Foster P.	Hamilton V.
Close E.	Davies S.	Fox S.	Handel K.
Clunie M.	Davies V.	Franklin R.	Handscombe D.
Cockley G.	Daw D.	Fraser R.A.	Hanley A.M.
Cocks A.	Dawe S.	Fryer P.	Harkness D.
Cody J.	Dawson A.	Furley D.	Harrad R.
Coen L.	Dickie G.	Gallifent M.	Harris E.
Coffey W.	Dickinson B.	Gareze C.	Harris K.
Cole H.L.	Dickson M.	Garner A.	Harris M.
Cole J.	Dixon D.	Garrett P.	Harrison B.
Coleman A.	Djaezari B.	Garstin I.	Hartley J.
Collings S.	Dobie S.	Gee W.	Harvey L.
Collins V.P.	Dorling R.	Gell I.	Hayton R.
Colyer J.	Douglas J.	Getgood M.	Heafield S.
Connolly J.D.R.	Douglas-Jones A.G.	Gilbert C.	Hegarty F.
Connolly L.	Dover H.	Gilbert D.	Helme D.
Cook A.	Drabu Y.	Gill G.	Henderson D.C.
Cooke A.	Dransfield D.	Gillett M.B.	Henderson J.
Coombe J.	Dundas S.A.C.	Gilligan M.	Hendy S.
Coombes S.	Dyer J.A.	Gilroy D.	Henry J.
Cooper H.	Dziewulski P.	Goddard G.	Herbert P.
Copeland G.P.	Easto J.	Goddard M.	Hewlett M.
Corbishley C.M.	Eaton S.	Gooch H.	Heyworth N.
Cornelius E.	Edwards K.	Gooday P.	Higgins J.

Higgs S.	Jordan-Moss J.	Lyons C.B.A.	Morley T.
Hillocks P.	Jowett C.	Mackenzie H.	Morris A.
Hinwood E.	Keddie L.	MacKenzie I.	Morrison B.
Hippsley C.	Keean S.	Mackersie A.	Mulvey S.
Hobbs L.	Kendall L.	Madders D.J.	Murdoch J.
Hock Y.L.	Kenyon S.	Mahy N.J.	Murrell D.
Hodgkins D.	Kenyon W.E.	Mann G.	Nana A.
Hoff R.	Kerrigan G.	Manser M.	Nash R.
Hogan A.	Kerringan G.	Marriage R.	Nash S.
Holden J.	Kesseler G.	Martin J.	Naylor K.
Holland N.	Khalid Z.	Masamha S.	Nee P.
Holliday V.	Kilpatrick E.	Masters P.	Needham S.
Holmes W.	King M.	Mawdesley W.P.	Nelson G.
Horne J.	King S.L.	Mayers M.	Newman T.
Houghton I.	Kirton C.B.	Mayover K.	Newton K.
Houlahan J.	Klein L.	McAfee A.	Nice G.
Howgrave-Graham P.	Knott J.	McArdle A.	Nicholson R.W.
Hughes R.G.	Kondratowicz G.	McCleane G.	Norman G.
Hull J.	Kuczyc R.	McCormack P.A.	Norman J.
Humphreys T.	Lacey V.	McCoy J.	North R.
Hunt C.M.	Lamb D.	McCullagh L.	Norton J.
Hunter B.	Lane R.	McGarvey D.	O'Dowd J.J.
Hurn N.	Lasky A.	McIlroy B.	O'Driscoll P.
Hurren K.	Last N.	Mckay K.	Offord J.
Hutchings L.	Latham S.	McKenzie I.	Okoli U.
Ince M.	Lawson A.H.	McLean J.G.M.	Orrin L.
Ince S.	Le May C.	McLoughlan L.	Otter S.
Ismaili N.	Leake J.	McMullen C.	Oyede C.
Jack L.	Leeson E.	McPherson C.	Pace C.
Jackson A.M.	Leow T.	Melville Jones G.R.	Palmer U.
Jackson E.	Letcher G.M.	Mendham B.	Park J.
Jackson M.	Lewis B.	Mercer J.	Parker M.
Jalloh S.S.	Lewis C.	Mercer N.	Parker N.
Jennings J.	Lewis E.	Merrill A.	Parker S.
Jennings M.	Lewis M.	Middleton M.	Parkins J.
Jessup M.	Liggitt J.	Milan S.	Parry A.
Joglekar V.M.	Linnett A.	Milhench M.	Parsons S.
Johnston J.	Lister A.	Miller M.	Patel K.
Johri S.	Lloyd-Davies S.	Milne S.	Paterson H.
Jones E.M.	Longan M.A.	Missons H.	Peachey M.
Jones G.	Longson J.	Mitchell N.	Peake A.
Jones H.	Loseby V.	Mitze M.	Pearce L.
Jones J.A.	Lott M.F.	Mohamid W.	Pearce P.
Jones L.	Lowe D.	Moore A.	Pearson J.
Jones P.	Lund T.	Moore J.	Perkins K.
Jones S.	Lynch C.	Morgan A.	Peters W.M.
Jones V.	Lyons C.	Morkane T.	Phillip G.

Phillips R.
Pinder S.
Poole G.
Power C.
Power V.
Pratt M.
Priest R.
Prouse T.
Punter A.
Pyne D.
Pyper P.C.
Quickmire S.
Rampson D.
Ramsay K.
Ramsay S.
Rankin M.
Rao M.
Rashid M.
Rawling J.
Record E.
Redfern L.
Redmayne A.
Rees A.M.
Reeves R.
Reeves S.
Rice A.
Riddell J.
Riesewyk C.
Riley J.
Rix F.
Robinson K.N.
Robson L.
Rogers B.
Rooney J.
Rosenberg I.L.
Ross A.H.
Ross L.D.
Rushmer J.
Russell I.
Ryan P.
Ryan S.
Salmon I.
Salmon J.
Salmons N.
Scammell N.
Scott K.
Sergi C.

Serginson L.
Sewell P.
Shannon A.
Sharp E.
Sharp J.
Shaw J.
Sheffield E.A.
Shelley A.
Shenkorov A.
Sheridan P.
Shilton D.
Shiner V.
Shirley Y.
Shuttleworth T.
Sides C.A.
Sidhu K.
Sildown D.J.
Simmonds G.
Simmons E.
Simpson A.
Simpson K.
Simpson R.
Sister Bernadette Marie
Slaney W.
Sleight J.
Small N.
Smith C.
Smith J.
Smith J.L.
Smith L.
Smith R.
Smooker S.
Snowball D.
Spencer I.
Stacey S.
Stamp G.W.H.
Stanley P.
Stebbings P.
Steer D.
Stellon P.
Stephenson J.
Stevens G.
Stewart A.
Stewart E.
Stimson M.
Stock D.
Stocker C.

Stoker S.
Stone C.
Stoner M.
Storey N.
Strahan K.
Stratton A.
Stretton J.
Stride P.C.
Stroud M.
Suarez V.
Summers L.
Sutton S.
Suvarna S.K.
Swabey C.
Tanner P.
Taylor A.
Taylor J.
Taylor P.
Taylor Z.
Temple L.
Terry G.
Tett L.
Thickett A.
Thomas A.
Thomas S.
Thompson R.
Thomson G.
Thorpe L.
Tingay T.
Tubbs J.
Tucker I.
Turnbull L.
Turner J.
Turner P.
Tuzzio L.
Tyrer S.
Ugar A.
Uraiby J.A.H.
Valle J.
Van Someren V.
Vasudev K.S.
Verrow S.
Vince J.
Vincent J.
Vincent S.
Vine G.
Vleugels M.

Vognsen M.
Walker R.
Walley D.
Walmsley M.
Walton J.
Ward C.
Ward J.
Ward P.J.
Ward R.
Wareham S.
Wark K.
Warner K.
Washington K.
Watson P.
Way L.
Weaver R.M.
Webster D.
Webster G.
Weir C.
Welsh A.
Wharton N.
Whitcombe M.
White S.
Whitmore J.
Whittam J.
Wilding J.
Wilkie C.
Wilkinson D.
Wilkinson L.
Williams A.R.
Williams C.
Williams G.
Williams H.
Williams H.
Williams L.
Wilner G.
Wilson C.
Witton C.
Wood H.
Wood N.
Woodyer A.
Wotton D.
Wright C.
Young M.